VITAL CONVERSATIONS

VITAL CONVERSATIONS

IMPROVING

COMMUNICATION

BETWEEN DOCTORS

AND PATIENTS

DENNIS ROSEN, MD

COLUMBIA UNIVERSITY PRESS *NEW YORK*

Columbia University Press
Publishers Since 1893
New York   Chichester, West Sussex
cup.columbia.edu

Library of Congress Cataloging-in-Publication Data
Rosen, Dennis, 1967– author.
Vital conversations : improving communication between doctors and patients /
Dennis Rosen.
p. ; cm.
Includes bibliographical references and index.
ISBN 978-0-231-16444-3 (cloth : alk. paper) — ISBN 978-0-231-53804-6 (e-book)
I. Title
[DNLM: 1. Physician-Patient Relations. 2. Communications.
3. Patient Satisfaction. W 62]
R727.3
610.69'6—dc23
2014003433

Columbia University Press books are printed on permanent
and durable acid-free paper.

This book is printed on paper with recycled content.
Printed in the United States of America

c 10 9 8 7 6 5 4 3 2 1

Cover design: Mary Ann Smith

References to websites (URLs) were accurate at the time of writing.
Neither the author nor Columbia University Press is responsible for URLs
that may have expired or changed since the manuscript was prepared.

To Vered, Yuval, Hadas, and Avigail,
with much love, appreciation, and pride.

CONTENTS

ACKNOWLEDGMENTS

THIS BOOK could not have been written without the help of so many along the way.

First off, I would like to thank some of the many people who have enabled me to channel my passion for the written word and to make the transition from passive consumer into an active producer. Thank you to the editors at *Psychology Today* for giving me the opportunity to blog about pediatric sleep and other topics on their website. Thank you, too, to the editors at the various newspapers, magazines, and journals whose receptiveness to my writing in the forms of essays, op-ed pieces, and book reviews was key to encouraging me to persevere along this path: John Zeller at the *Journal of the American Medical Association*; Shelly Cohen at the *Boston Herald*; Mary Duenwald, Honor Jones, Sewell Chan, David Corcoran, Alex Star, and David Kelly at the *New York Times*; Nicole Lamy and Paul Makishima at the *Boston Globe*; Michael Todd and Tom Jacobs at the *Pacific Standard*; Barbara Sibbald at the *Canadian Medical Association Journal*; Lee Brown at the *Journal of Clinical Sleep Medicine*; and Elleke Bal and Babette Dunkelgrun at *Ode*.

Ethan, Molly, Liz, Donna, Alice, and Amy, whom I met at Grub Street in Boston—an outstanding resource for writers at any stage of their careers—helped me hone my writing and encouraged me to persevere even as the rejections kept coming in hard and fast. A big *Thank*

You to all of you: your insight and guidance along the way have been invaluable. Likewise, I am grateful to my colleagues at Boston Children's Hospital, who have been extremely supportive of my writing. I owe special words of thanks to Craig Gerard, whose support of my decision to pursue my writing has been solid and unwavering, and to Donna Giromini, who has cheered me on from the very beginning.

Thank you to Julie Silver, editor of books at Harvard Health Publications, who has taught me so much about writing and publishing.

I am exceedingly grateful to Patrick Fitzgerald, Bridget Flannery-McCoy, Kathryn Schell, Michael Haskell, and Robert Fellman, my editors at Columbia University Press. Your guidance, coaching, suggestions, and skillful editing from start to finish made this a much better book than I could ever possibly have hoped to write on my own.

I am also very grateful to my parents, Meredith and Lewis Rosen; my brother, Jonathan Rosen; and my sister, Amy Lutnick, for all of their love and support, as well as to my mother- and father-in-law, Ruchama and Leslie Leiserowitz. I wish we all lived closer to one another. Yuval, Hadas, and Avigail: you're wonderful kids, and I feel truly blessed to have you in my life. And to my lovely wife, Vered, whose support and encouragement throughout this whole process have been key to being able to develop my writing to where it is today (not least of which includes letting me disappear for hours into my own private space on weekends and evenings): thank you, thank you, thank you! I never could have done this without you.

I am very grateful to my many teachers and mentors along the way who have taught me through example about how important good communication with patients is to the healing process. Special words of thanks go to Levana Sinai, my department chief in Pediatrics B at Kaplan Medical Center, and to the late Mary Ellen Beck Wohl, former head of the Division of Respiratory Diseases at Boston Children's Hospital. I'd also like to thank my mentors and teachers at the Institute for Professionalism and Ethical Practice at Boston Children's Hospital—Elaine Meyer, Bob Truog, Stephen Brown, David Browning, and Elizabeth Rider—for sharing so generously of your time, experiences, expertise, and insight. Thank you, too, for allowing me to participate in several of the institute's workshops while writing this book: they were an invaluable experience that I wish every clinician were fortunate enough to experience.

Another big thank you to the many people who have read portions of this book and provided me with valuable feedback along the way: Bridget Flannery-McCoy; Patrick Fitzgerald; the anonymous reviewers of the proposal and manuscript in its various forms and iterations; my wife, Vered; my parents; my brother, Jonathan; Molly Howes; Donna Luff; Amy Faeskorn; Liz Quinn; Alice Harkness; Rhonda Roumani; Ethan Gilsdorf; David Patterson; Levana Sinai; Orna Flidel; Sharon Alzner; Michael Todd; Elaine Meyer; Denise Anderson; Debra Boyer; David Browning; Peter Weinstock; Laura Hornbrook; Donna Giromini; and Craig Gerard. Thank you, too, to the parents of two of the children described within the pages of this book, Isabelle and Sally, and to Sally as well, who read, made very helpful suggestions about, and gave their blessings for the segments that relate to them to be published. Although I am not able to publish their names, I am very grateful to them for their graciousness and help.

And finally, last but certainly not least, an especially big *Thank You* to my patients and their families, who have taught me so much over the years. Even though I still may not always get it right, you are the reason I keep trying to get better at my own communication skills. You are the reason I view improving my abilities in this area—as well as those of other physicians—as one of the most important and fulfilling lifelong tasks ahead of me.

AUTHOR'S NOTE

THE MEDICAL information provided within this book is general in nature, and in no way should it be understood as medical advice. This book cannot replace a face-to-face consultation with a qualified medical professional.

The identities of all of the patients and their families as well as of most of the physicians have been altered in order to protect their privacy. This includes changes made to names, genders, dates, places, and diseases. The only people who were named (and with permission) are Ms. Denise Anderson and Drs. Mary Ellen Beck Wohl, Levana Sinai, and Orna Flidel. All of the stories herein did in fact occur and are presented to the best of my recollection, subject to the caveats above.

A portion of chapter 1 was published in somewhat different form as "Changing Parental Attitudes on Child Vaccinations," *Pacific Standard* (April 18, 2012), http://www.psmag.com/health/changing-parental -attitudes-on-child-vaccinations-41350/.

The epigraph to chapter 6 is reprinted with permission of Open Court Publishing Company, a division of Carus Publishing Company, Chicago, Ill. It is taken from Thomas Stephen Szasz, *The Untamed Tongue: A Dissenting Dictionary* (Chicago: Open Court, 1990).

VITAL CONVERSATIONS

1

BETTER OUTCOMES, LOWER COSTS

It is the province of knowledge to speak,
and it is the privilege of wisdom to listen.

—Oliver Wendell Holmes, American physician, 1809–1894

THE FIRST, and so far only, time I was hospitalized was when I was eighteen and had become dehydrated a few days after developing a relapse of mononucleosis. Soon after my arrival at Rambam Hospital in the northern Israeli city of Haifa, I began to develop ulcers inside my mouth. These soon spread to cover my gums and inner cheeks and were exquisitely painful. By the end of my second day there, I was unable to drink or eat anything.

I was weak, in a lot of pain, and utterly demoralized. I had been battling mono for the previous six weeks, and as if that weren't enough, now this!

On rounds the next day, my mouth was the focus of everyone's attention. Although I had been given lidocaine gel to numb it up, I could feel my cheeks being stretched tautly against the gloved fingers poking around inside my mouth. My lips were being turned inside out and prized away from the gums to expose better the sores within. Close to a dozen people were rounding on me that day, and I had not the faintest idea who most of them were. Still, I was confident that they would be able to figure out why I was in such discomfort and help me get better.

As the last set of fingers slid slowly out of my mouth with a thick strand of blood-tinged saliva in tow, the most senior-looking man in the group turned toward the door and walked slowly in its direction. He said something in a mixture of Hebrew and Latin that I wasn't able to understand. The others nodded, and began to follow him out of the room.

"Doctor," I called after him, my numbed-up tongue and lips making the words difficult to articulate. "What's wrong with me?"

He hesitated at the doorway, rested his hand on the door handle, and turned his head back toward me. "Gingivitis," he answered.

I had never heard that word before and didn't know what it meant. I certainly didn't like the way it sounded. All of a sudden, I was very frightened and felt small and inexplicably ashamed, unworthy even. Instead of asking what gingivitis was and why I had gotten it, I asked about its treatment.

"Keep on rinsing your mouth with salt water, and use the lidocaine gel for pain."

"How long will it take until I'm better?" I asked.

He shrugged his shoulders silently and turned away. Before I even realized it, he and the others were gone. I was now alone, my mind racing as I wondered in terror what this gingivitis was, why I had been stricken by it, and whether it would indeed ever go away.

It took about a week until the sores in my mouth had fully healed. I still don't know exactly what caused them. Most likely they were the result of a secondary viral infection that had overwhelmed my weakened immune system, but at this point, it doesn't really matter.

What does matter, however, is that the anxiety and stress that I experienced that morning remain stamped in my memory with an intensity that refuses to recede, despite the passing of more than a quarter-century. It didn't have to be that way. If only that particular physician or anyone else from the group had taken the time to explain to me that gingivitis merely meant inflammation of the gums and that this was a self-limited condition that, although unpleasant and uncomfortable, would pass within a few days, my response would have been altogether different. But that wasn't something they seemed conscious of needing to do. It was as if they saw themselves as charged solely with tending to my physical needs, with any others I may have had being outside their purview.

Since then I've had many opportunities to reflect upon that week I spent in the hospital, within the context of my regular interactions with my own patients and their families in my present role as a pediatric pulmonologist. I believe that my experiences then have made me a better physician today than I might otherwise have become.

Even now, whenever I find myself displaced from my usual role of physician into that of patient, I gain new insight into aspects of my practice that I had never previously considered. Becoming a patient has the sobering effect of causing me to reflect upon some of my own actions as a physician that had previously seemed appropriate and effective to me but that in hindsight appear woefully inadequate. I become much more aware of how I interact with my own patients and their families and resolve to do better in ways that I previously had been completely oblivious to, despite having worked with patients, first as a nurse during medical school and then as a physician, for more than twenty years now.

Good communication between physicians and patients is vitally important to the well-being of patients, as it is to physicians, the health-care system, and society as a whole. Good communication establishes the trust necessary for patients to open up to their physicians and to commit themselves to the healing process prescribed by their physicians. As I will discuss in chapter 2, this process of healing extends far beyond the chemical effects of the medications and the physical results of the surgeries themselves. Good communication between physicians and patients leads to greater satisfaction for both, more frequent use of preventive medical services, and better adherence by patients to treatment plans. Not only do these improve health outcomes; they save money as well.

Over the last decade, a convergence of market forces, economic realities, and renewed political will to address the myriad problems plaguing health-care provision in this country has brought about broad changes in how medicine is and will be practiced, now and in the years ahead. Change is inevitable because of the ever-increasing and ultimately unsustainable cost of health care, which currently consumes almost 18 percent of GDP, or $2.5 trillion annually.[1] As if that weren't bad enough, the Institute of Medicine estimates that approximately 30 percent of health-care spending in the United States, more than $765 billion *each year*, is wasted, the result of unnecessary or inefficiently delivered services, excessive administrative costs, and missed prevention opportunities.[2]

There is absolutely no disputing the need to control and, ultimately, to reduce spending on health care if we want the American economy to thrive. My concern, however, based upon trends that I've witnessed and lived through since I first began my medical studies in 1988, is that many of the proposals to control health-care costs fail to consider just how fundamental good communication between patients and physicians is to the good *and* efficient practice of medicine. Without attending to this extremely important aspect of health-care provision, these proposals will disappoint as far as improving health outcomes and reducing costs go, to the detriment of everyone involved. As I will show, interventions that maintain and improve the quality of communication between physicians and patients can and do result in better outcomes and in significant cost savings.

This is why I have written this book. My goal is to convince you of the absolute importance of good communication between physicians and patients, to encourage you to think about how you can make each physician-patient interaction you take part in a better one, and to provide you with guidance about how to do that. This is especially important if you are a physician or are in training to become one. The same is true for nurse practitioners and physician assistants and, perhaps to a lesser degree, other allied health professionals. However, regardless of whether you are a patient, potential patient, or physician, I hope that this book will help you understand why this issue is so important to you. I also hope that it will lead you to become an active participant in a public conversation that needs to take place and that will lead to the implementation of strategies that preserve, nurture, and enhance good communication between physicians and patients, to the benefit of us all.

Throughout this book, *patient* will refer to anyone voluntarily seeking—or involuntarily brought by others to receive—medical care because of a perceived condition of poor health, objective or subjective in nature. Likewise, *physician* will refer to a person who has undergone recognized training in biomedicine and has been authorized by society to practice it, without restriction, in the medical or surgical realm.

One more thing: because the balance of power in the relationship between patient and physician is so heavily skewed toward the physician, I have chosen to refer to the communication between the two as *physician-patient* communication instead of as *patient-physician* communication. I have done this in order to signify where I feel the onus of improving this communication lies: on physicians. This is true even though patients vastly outnumber physicians, are the raison d'être for these relationships, and stand to gain the most from their improvement.

Regardless of a person's usual social station, upon the simple act of seeking medical care because of a perceived condition of poor health, the patient enters into a rigidly hierarchical world within which much of his autonomy is relinquished. As Bonnie Blair O'Connor of Brown Medical School writes in her foreword to Chloë Atkins's book *My Imaginary Illness*: "Many of us have . . . felt frightened, ignored, belittled, accused, dismissed, or deeply and painfully humiliated by healthcare professionals on whose knowledge, skills, and mercy we have depended when we were sick."[3]

The balance of power between patient and physician is tilted heavily in favor of the latter: the patient, after all, is the one seeking help in alleviating discomfort, disability, disfigurement, or death. The physician, however, is not in most cases at personal risk from the patient's disease and possesses the knowledge to relieve and perhaps even remedy the patient's condition. The patient may have only one shot at beating his disease and no recourse other than to enlist a physician's assistance to do so. Although patients are usually free to select their specific physicians, they remain dependent upon *a* physician for treatment. The physician, however, can rest secure in the knowledge that, barring egregious malpractice or negligence on his part, there will always be more patients lining up at his door.

This imbalance of power leaves the patient with few choices: to accept what the physician proposes to overcome the disease; to reject it outright; or to seek help from another physician or healer, biomedical or spiritual, who may or may not be available. While this imbalance becomes obvious to anyone upon assuming the role of patient, it is not always at the forefront of the physician's awareness. Indeed, it is often only when the physician (or one of her family members) becomes a patient herself that it is fully appreciated. This is the theme of Randa Haines's 1991 movie *The Doctor*, in which an arrogant cardiothoracic surgeon is diagnosed with cancer. His experiences as a patient, especially the memorable interaction he has with the detached and cold otolaryngologist who first gives him his diagnosis, cause him to transform into a much more sympathetic and empathetic physician by the end of the film.

PLAN OF THE BOOK

In this first chapter, I'll make the case for why good communication between physician and patient is so important and how its promotion and enhancement can lead to a better and more efficient healthcare system. As I'll show, the improved outcomes and reduced costs stemming from better communication are achieved through improved medical adherence, decreased medical error and rehospitalization rates, reduced malpractice claims, and higher physician satisfaction. Chapter 2 will discuss the advantages of tailoring medical care to meet the needs of the patient in accordance with his or her values and preferences, in real time as well as through advance planning. It will also explore the inherent therapeutic effect of the physician-patient relationship, what the physician and psychoanalyst Michael Balint refers to as the "drug 'doctor,'"[4] as exemplified by the placebo effect.

Chapter 3 will look at how differences in culture, belief systems, and disease conceptualization can undermine the ability of physician and patient to establish a meaningful dialogue and to construct a satisfactory relationship. Chapters 4 and 5 will explore the importance of the physician's not merely treating the patient's disease but also attending to her *illness* (the patient's response to disease) and *sickness* (society's response to the patient and her disease and the roles this casts upon her). Chapter 5 will also discuss the role of communication-skills training for physicians in improving these capabilities. Chapter 6 will examine how bias and stigma on the part of physicians, as well as socioeconomic and health-literacy disparities between physicians and their patients, can interfere with effective communication.

Chapter 7 will identify ways of improving physician-patient communication at a systems level, through the strategic use of medical decision-making aids, health-information technology, and better health-care-facility design. Chapter 8 will provide practical suggestions to both patients and physicians on how to improve communication in the one-on-one health interactions that they participate in. It will conclude with a description of ways in which the health-promoting effects of the direct interaction between the physician and the patient can be extended into the pre- and postvisit segments of the medical encounter and beyond so as to improve its efficiency and provide more long-lasting value. This is, in essence, a counterargument to those whose calculations of efficiency, based upon the absolute number of patients seen by a physician within a certain number of minutes, ignore the true measures of value: better health outcomes and reduced overall costs.

THE IMPORTANCE TO PATIENTS OF GOOD PHYSICIAN-PATIENT COMMUNICATION

Some of the most intimate conversations we will ever have are with our physicians. With them, we talk about our struggles with the loss of our health and what it brings: pain, disability, and an unsparing perspective on our own inevitable mortality. Hoping to keep these at bay, we discuss and negotiate with our physicians whether to pursue painful or disabling treatments or surgeries or to forgo certain pleasurable activities that until recently we took for granted. With our physicians we share some of our deepest hopes—and darkest fears—about ourselves and our loved ones.

Trust lies at the foundation of the relationships we have with our physicians. Fundamentally, we must be able to believe that they are dedicated to preserving and restoring our health and to alleviating our discomfort. For this trust to be established and maintained, good bidirectional communication—expressive and receptive—must exist between physician and patient. We want our physicians to treat us with respect, empathy, and compassion. We also need them to be competent and ethical, to possess integrity, and to be committed to providing us with unwaveringly excellent care. With the exception of professional competence, however, the only way we can judge whether a physician possesses these attributes is by how she or he communicates them directly to us.

Most people, especially when finding themselves in the role of patient, recognize how important good communication with their physicians is to their own well-being. In one survey, 95 percent of adults ranked bedside manner and communication skills as the key determinants when choosing a physician.[5] Yet in all too many medical interactions, patients note that these elements are conspicuously absent. One large study of American adults conducted by the Commonwealth Fund found that more than 25 percent reported that their physicians didn't encourage them to ask questions. Thirty percent described not receiving clear instructions from their physicians regarding what symptoms to watch out for or when to seek further care or treatment, and almost 40 percent said that their physicians didn't always discuss different treatment options or involve them in medical decision making.[6]

Physicians, too, recognize the importance of good communication with their patients, even when not always successful at it. Researchers who interviewed a large group of primary-care physicians found that the degree to which the physicians perceived the quality of their interactions with their patients as "positive" had the strongest effect on their career satisfaction, greater even than income.[7]

Good communication between patient and physician is essential for the physician to be able to recognize and appropriately treat the problems that bring the patient to see him in the first place.[8] This should come as no surprise since it is difficult for physicians to successfully treat something they are unaware of. In medical school I was taught that 80 percent of the diagnosis could be made by taking a good history from the patient, with another 10 percent gleaned from the physical examination. This, it turns out, is no mere aphorism.[9] The subjective history supplied by the patient provides the context within which objective data collected by the physician are assessed and directs the physician's focus to those matters that require his attention.

A good medical history proves to be important even when the presence of objective abnormalities on the physical examination should ostensibly suffice for the physician to start treatment, irrespective of whether the patient complains about them. This was demonstrated by a large study that followed more than 7,100 patients whose blood pressure was found to be elevated upon routine measurement when visiting their physicians in their offices. Those patients who had identified their hypertension as the reason for their visits were twice as likely to be treated for it as those who hadn't.[10] This is a striking finding because the untreated hypertension posed an increased risk of heart disease and stroke for all of them, as their physicians presumably knew, and should have prompted treatment irrespective of whether the patients had discussed their blood pressure.

THE CONNECTION BETWEEN GOOD PHYSICIAN-PATIENT COMMUNICATION AND MEDICAL ADHERENCE

The physician's task does not end with the diagnosis of disease and the prescription of treatment. No less an important—and in many instances the most difficult—part of his role is to find ways of getting his patients to adhere to the treatment plans he develops with and for them. This is especially true for patients with chronic disease, but it is also a problem in the acute-disease setting as well, in both children and adults.[11]

Joyce Cramer of the Yale University School of Medicine has defined medical adherence as "the extent to which a patient acts in accordance with the prescribed interval and dose of a dosing regimen [prescribed by a health-care professional]."[12] There is a robust body of evidence correlating better communication between physicians and patients with improved medical adherence.[13] This is true for many reasons. Better physician-patient communication tends to result in patients assuming a more active and participatory role in medical-decision making, and leads to increased patient trust in the physician. Both promote increased patient willingness to carry out physicians' recommendations, in both the outpatient and inpatient care settings.[14]

It's hard to overstate just how important patient trust in the physician is for good medical adherence. Some studies have found that negative patient attitudes toward physicians are more highly associated with medical nonadherence than the presence of side effects from the medications or their cost.[15] For example, patients with mood disorders have reported that more "collaborative" physician communication styles improved both their satisfaction and subsequent adherence with the antidepressant medications they were prescribed. The same connection between patient trust in physicians and medical adherence has been documented in other chronic diseases as well, such as hypertension and diabetes.[16]

Better patient-physician communication leads to improved understanding by the patient of the disease processes in need of treatment, what the treatments being prescribed are intended to accomplish, their possible side effects, and how and when the treatments should be administered or taken.[17] This last point is particularly important. Some medications, after all, are prescribed in order to *relieve* symptoms and should only be taken if and when symptoms occur, such as ibuprofen when prescribed to relieve fever or headache. Alternatively, other medications are prescribed to be taken regularly, *even in the absence of symptoms*. For example: antihypertensive medications that are prescribed to treat high blood pressure precisely to *prevent* the emergence of symptoms. If the patient does not understand the difference, he is liable to overtreat or undertreat himself, leading to poorer outcomes because of side effects from the medications or complications from disease flare-ups or progression. This can happen even though the patient believes that he is doing exactly as his physician instructed him.

The cost of medications can and often does affect patients' willingness to take them. However, lowering patients' out-of-pocket expenses—by reducing copayments for example—has been shown to be less effective at increasing medical adherence than improving patients' comprehension of how to take their medications, why they even need to take them, and the potential side effects they may encounter.[18] Still, when there's just not enough money and the patient needs to choose between buying food or medicine, the choice isn't difficult, especially if the patient isn't convinced that the medication is truly necessary. And, indeed, the decision to forgo the treatment can seem justified when no immediate consequences, such as the reemergence of symptoms, are seen or felt.

Not being able to afford the cost of medications can be embarrassing for patients. One study found that almost 40 percent of medically nonadherent patients, for whom the cost of medications was the driving factor behind their nonadherence, had not discussed this with their physicians.[19] Over the years I have been asked by many parents whether I could prescribe a less expensive but equally effective medication to control their child's asthma and have tried my best to do so. Yet I am sure that there were many others who did not raise the issue and who wound up not giving their children what I had prescribed because of the cost, unbeknownst to me. Unless discussed, it may not even occur to the physician to try to find a less expensive substitute treatment, and the patient will continue to simply not take the medication that has been prescribed.

The scope of medical nonadherence is vast. A recent review of the health-care claims of more than 706,000 adults being treated for at least one of seven chronic diseases found rates of medical nonadherence ranging between 32 and 63 percent, depending on the specific disease.[20] For the purposes of that study, nonadherent patients were defined as those who hadn't taken their medications as prescribed for more than 20 percent of the first year in which they were prescribed.

Medical nonadherence is a problem for many reasons. As Dr. C. Everett Koop, the former surgeon general of the United States famously said, "Drugs don't work in patients who don't take them."[21] Not only do nonadherent patients not get better; they often get sicker as their diseases continue to progress unchecked. This was the unsurprising conclusion of a large study that reviewed the medical records of more than 49,000 patients with high blood pressure who were enrolled in the Tennessee Medicaid program over a seven-year period. Just as you might expect, those patients who did not fill their prescriptions were more likely to suffer stroke or death than those who did. Overall, it is estimated that approximately 125,000 Americans die each year because of medical nonadherence.[22]

As obvious as this may seem, it's worth repeating: *If you're sick and don't take your medications, you are more likely to get sicker and die sooner than if you do.* The proven benefits of biomedicine in many aspects of health maintenance and restoration are precisely why it remains in such high demand and why we spend so much on it, individually and collectively.

In addition to being healthier, medically adherent patients also generally wind up consuming less-expensive care. For example, patients who are not medically adherent have fewer office-based visits with their physicians and more emergency-room visits and hospitalizations than those who are. From the perspectives of the health-care system and society—which ultimately pays the bills—the cost savings is clear. Emergency-room visits are more than 4.5 times as expensive as office-based visits, and each day spent in the hospital is ten times more expensive than an office visit. It has been calculated that in 2010 alone, the total *direct* costs of medical nonadherence for just three conditions, diabetes, hypertension, and dyslipidemia (high cholesterol), exceeded $105 billion.[23]

Another problem with poor medical adherence is that many medications lose their effectiveness when not taken properly. For example, bacteria can become resistant to antibiotics that are not taken consistently. This not only puts the patient at risk of becoming overwhelmed by infection but also makes the entire community more vulnerable since those antibiotics can no longer be relied upon to treat the resistant bugs effectively. Poor and inconsistent adherence to therapy is one of the main reasons for the emergence of extremely resistant and dangerous forms of tuberculosis that not only pose a major public-health hazard globally but are also costly to control. The eradication of one outbreak of multi-drug-resistant tuberculosis in New York City in the early 1990s, for example, is estimated to have cost one billion dollars.[24]

There is no question that physicians need to be more active in discussing medication adherence with their patients. This was demonstrated by a study in which primary-care medical visits were videotaped and analyzed. The researchers found that the physicians asked only basic questions about fewer than one-third of their patients' medications and really only delved into the issue of nonadherence for 4.3 percent of them. This is important because only half of the nonadherent patients actually volunteered that information to their physicians on their own.[25]

The implication is clear: without effectively soliciting information about medical nonadherence, physicians cannot take the extra steps necessary to help their patients become more adherent. The care their patients receive becomes suboptimal, thereby increasing the risk of complications as well as incurring the additional and wholly avoidable medical costs associated with treating them.

WHEN PATIENTS ARE NOT FULLY OPEN WITH THEIR PHYSICIANS

There is also the delicate issue of incomplete truthfulness, or less-than-full disclosure, on the part of patients. This happens more than one might think. Not necessarily because patients are purposely trying to deceive their physicians or are trying to wheedle something out of them—although that happens, too, especially when disability compensation is involved. Instead, patients may not be completely honest with their physicians because they're trying to convince themselves that *this* time things are going to be different. This time, they are serious, and there's really no point in dwelling on their fallen past: *I have no clue where those extra twenty pounds came from; I'm only eating 1,500 calories a day and working out five times a week. It's not because I haven't been watching what I eat: I've not so much as looked at a single carb all of the last month* (unspoken is the obvious: the calories didn't just materialize out of thin air). Another is wishful thinking: *Maybe if I ignore x, it will go away on its own.*

Openness in conversations between physician and patient allows information to surface that then enables the physician to provide guidance to the patient about avoiding conditions that, though not yet present, may still pose a risk to the patient, for example, the acquisition of a sexually transmitted disease by adolescents through unprotected sex or the long-term health risks of obesity. Without anticipatory guidance, there is greater likelihood that these will metamorphose from potential to actual problems. Not only will the patient's health be affected adversely, but additional costs will be borne by the health-care system, costs that might possibly have been avoided altogether.

Patients may avoid discussing their problems with their physicians because of denial, shame, or perceived stigma, which I'll discuss in greater detail in chapter 6. For example, a woman who comes in for an annual checkup may not volunteer that she suffers from domestic violence unless specifically asked about her home environment in a way that enables her to provide an honest answer. Patients may simply hold back on volunteering certain information to their physicians if they fear that this may result in their being judged negatively. This is especially true when it comes to poor medical adherence.

If you were to ask most people what they think about someone who consults a physician about how to become healthy, disregards that advice, and then returns—to the same physician!—for another consultation because she still hasn't gotten better, they'd tell you she's crazy. It really makes no sense to waste one's time, and that of a physician, if there is no intention of following his advice. Still, it happens all too often.

A recent study of almost six hundred patients enrolled in a program to quit smoking at the Department of Veterans Affairs' health system found that more than 20 percent of those who had claimed to have stopped smoking continued, nonetheless, to have high levels of cotinine, a metabolite of nicotine secreted into the urine of tobacco smokers—clear evidence that they were, in fact, continuing to smoke. A similar study in Scotland looked at the prevalence of unreported smoking in more than 3,400 pregnant Scottish women. There, too, it was found that 25 percent more women had cotinine in their urine than had admitted to smoking.[26] Perhaps this can be attributed to the social stigma attached to smoking while pregnant because of the harm it is known to cause the developing fetus. It might also have represented a hope of turning over a new leaf: *Last night was my last cigarette, I swear.* Regardless, had their physicians been aware that these women were in fact continuing to smoke, they might have been more aggressive about getting them into smoking-cessation programs, thus sparing at least some of them—and their unborn children—the consequences.

I became acutely aware of this phenomenon after starting physical therapy for a back injury that left me with two herniated discs and unable to stand up or lie down straight without severe pain for three months. In addition to a slew of medications I had been prescribed to control pain and inflammation, I was given a regimen of back exercises by my physical therapist, Caitlyn. I did these exercises religiously every day and believe to this day that they were the only thing that helped me heal faster. Caitlyn was a knowledgeable and dedicated young woman who really knew what she was doing. Each time we met, she would teach me new exercises to strengthen my lumbar and abdominal muscles. I was especially impressed by how she used ultrasound to show me precisely which muscles I needed to tense up with each particular exercise. She was also beautiful and utterly charming.

I did exactly what Caitlyn told me to do, as she told me, and when she told me. I was a model patient, not least because I could feel the efforts translating into less pain and more function. Alas, the healing process was slow and long, and for almost ten full weeks I continued to require painkillers at night simply to be able to lie down.

That wasn't what I told Caitlyn, however, when she'd ask me how I was feeling each time we met.

"Much better," I'd reply, though my inability to straighten up fully was obvious.

"Are you still taking the narcotic pain relievers?" she'd ask, and I'd deny it, though it would still be several more weeks until I no longer needed them.

I felt stupid lying to her, especially since she could easily see that I was still limited in what I was able to do because of the pain, but I also couldn't bear to disappoint her. She was trying her best to help me, and I hated to let her down and have her think badly of me. That was when it dawned on me that many of my patients probably stretch the truth with me as well, even though I'm nowhere near as cute as Caitlyn. This experience taught me to probe deeply into the issue of adherence with my patients, especially with those whose response to the treatments I had prescribed wasn't what I had expected or hoped for. I learned that I needed to do this to find out if they, too, might be trying to shield me from unpleasant truths. It is, after all, simple human nature not to want to disappoint the person who seems to be trying so hard to help you for your own sake, not hers, and to have her think less of you as a result.

PATIENTS FAILING TREATMENT VERSUS TREATMENTS FAILING PATIENTS

Many physicians describe patients as "failing treatment" when the anticipated results are not achieved. This can be cancer that fails to go into remission, a bone infection that fails to respond to a prescribed course of antibiotics, or a pregnancy that doesn't materialize despite the use of powerful fertility drugs. A better way to describe this lack of success, however, is to say that the *treatment* has failed the *patient*. Although this distinction may sound purely semantic, it reminds us who—and what—serves whom. The treatment is intended and must therefore be tailored to help the patient and to meet his or her needs rather than being something for which the patient needs to turn his life upside-down and that will succeed only if the patient does his part. It also reminds physicians to consider those factors that are beyond the patient's control, such as genetic variability or the presence of other disease processes, that may interfere with the treatment's success.[27]

In some cases the patient's disease is amplified or made more difficult to treat effectively because of a second medical problem that the patient neglects to discuss with her physician, often because she doesn't connect the two. An example of this is untreated obstructive sleep apnea, which can in turn make diabetes much more difficult to control by altering the patient's metabolism and causing excessive daytime sleepiness that reduces her motivation to take her medications as prescribed. Another example is untreated depression, which significantly reduces medical adherence in patients with chronic diseases such as diabetes and AIDS.[28]

Sometimes, the urgency of treating a specific condition may seem so obvious to the physician that she may feel no need to discuss its implications with the patient, not realizing that the patient may actually perceive the problem as being much less significant. For example, the physician may want to start an asymptomatic patient with high blood pressure on medications to prevent complications such as heart disease and stroke. The patient, however, may not be aware of the potential risks that the untreated high blood pressure poses and be reluctant to take medicines that produce side effects while he continues to feel absolutely fine. Unless the physician tries to align the patient's conceptualization of the disease and the treatment plan with her own, there may be a significant gap in the patient's follow-through and adherence. The patient may pay lip service to carrying out the physician's recommendations and instructions while in reality having very little intention of following through with them.

Adherence with treatment can also be undermined for the opposite reason, namely, fear of the risks associated with the treatment, real or imagined: *I don't want my kids taking steroids for asthma; if they weren't dangerous, why would they have made such a big deal about them with Lance Armstrong?* In an article in *Cancer Nursing*, Carola Skott of the University of Göteborg quoted a patient with Hodgkin's disease who said: "I feel as though I have two enemies inside: one is the disease, one is the treatment that kills the tumor, but I fear that it will kill me first and after that the tumor."[29] This young woman's ambivalence about which of the two, treatment or disease, posed the greatest risk to her health is shared by many patients, even though most may refrain from voicing these fears to their physicians.

The easiest way for a physician to uncover gaps between how she and her patient perceive the risks of disease and the benefits of its treatment is to ask open-endedly about concerns regarding either of them. Not only can addressing these concerns help in the short term to reduce the patient's anxiety and allay his fears, some which may not be factually justified, but it is also likely to improve the patient's adherence with treatment in the medium and long terms as well.[30]

Some concerns are so terrifying that they are almost impossible for either the patient or her family to bring up, even when encouraged to. I have seen this many times with children who were referred to my pulmonary clinic because of an abnormal finding on a chest X ray or CT scan. Most times, these were simply the remnants of a previous infection, often one that neither the child nor his parents could remember as having been especially significant. When this was indeed the case, after taking a careful history and performing a thorough examination along with additional testing as needed, all that was needed was reassurance and a repeat imaging study a few months later to make sure that nothing had changed.

I cannot emphasize strongly enough how important *reassurance* is. Although lung cancer is extremely rare in the pediatric population, it is one of the most common forms of cancer in adults and certainly among the deadliest.[31] Many people have had firsthand experience with family members who have died from lung cancer, and because of this I make sure to stress to the family how rare it is in children, regardless of whether they have raised the question. And although in most cases the parents appear to be outwardly calm before I bring it up, many will break into tears of relief once I mention the "C-word" and explain to them that what their child has is almost certainly *not* cancer. This serves as a good reminder to me of the degree of anxiety that accompanies my patients and their parents on their visits with me and that, had I not looked for it, would have remained invisible to me. Without having discussed and defused their real concerns, one can only speculate as to the mental and physical toll these would have taken on the parents.

REDUCING ADVERSE EVENTS AND EARLY READMISSIONS FOLLOWING HOSPITAL DISCHARGE

Poor communication between physicians and patients is an important cause of readmission to the hospital shortly after being sent home. Many of these readmissions are caused by medication errors on the part of patients. Almost one out of every five Medicare patients sent home from the hospital winds up getting readmitted within thirty days of discharge. The annual cost to Medicare of these unanticipated hospitalizations is estimated to be $17.4 billion. To reduce this cost, the Hospital Readmissions Reduction Program was created as part of the Patient Protection and Affordable Care Act (a.k.a. Obamacare) and implemented in October 2012. This program mandates reduced payments by the Center for Medicare and Medicaid Services to hospitals with higher readmission rates than the national average for patients with comparable conditions.[32]

In general, patients are readmitted to the hospital shortly after discharge either because they were sent home too quickly (i.e., before they were really healthy enough to go home) or because recent changes to their medical management or health have overwhelmed their ability to care for themselves. In either case, the patient's condition rapidly deteriorates once he is back home and on his own, to the point where he soon requires additional care in a hospital setting.

It is interesting to note that the frequency of adverse events following discharge from the hospital, defined as unintended injury caused by the medical care itself, corresponds almost perfectly to the thirty-day readmission rate. Nineteen percent of patients experience post-discharge adverse events, and two-thirds of these involve medications, suggesting that better predischarge coaching and coordination might have prevented the majority of these.[33]

The findings of one study, in which forty-three English-speaking adult patients being discharged from a large academic hospital in New York were interviewed about their discharge medications and diagnoses, illustrate the scope of this problem. Eighty-six percent of the patients did not know what the common side effects of their medications were, 72 percent were unable to name all of their discharge medications—fewer than four, on average—and 63 percent did not understand why the medications had even been prescribed in the first place.[34] These are precisely the factors that predict good medical adherence, and if these findings are representative, it's surprising that readmission rates aren't higher still.

Consider a sixty-year-old man being discharged from the hospital following his first heart attack who now has to assimilate a whole raft of changes to his lifestyle and behavior to accommodate the limitations of his damaged heart. These might involve changing his diet; cutting back on or eliminating alcohol and tobacco consumption; giving up certain activities, such as sports or sexual activity; and aggressively pursuing weight loss. His heart attack may also have unmasked conditions that had been present for some time and of which he was unaware, such as hypertension or diabetes; it may also have triggered depression. These will also need to be treated. He may also need to start taking medications he is unfamiliar with and perhaps has never even heard of before. These medications may have side effects such as dizziness or lightheadedness that put him at risk of falling and injuring himself. He may decide simply to not take them, or he may take them incorrectly because he misunderstands the instructions he was given. Either way, he is at risk for complications that may shortly land him back in the hospital.

As noted earlier, whether a patient trusts her physician will determine the degree to which she is willing to follow the physician's treatment recommendations in the outpatient setting as well as upon discharge from the hospital. This is especially germane to the latter as care within the hospital is often provided not by the patient's regular physician, with whom she may have a longstanding relationship, but by physicians she has only just met and who are often assigned to her without her having any say in the matter. Complicating this is the fact that care teams, especially in academic hospitals, often include medical students and physicians in training (interns, residents, and fellows) who are constantly handing off care as they cycle on and off call. This is a recipe for confusion: one study found that 85 percent of patients admitted to a large academic hospital were unable to name the physician taking care of them correctly.[35] At the risk of stating the obvious: how could you possibly trust someone whose name you didn't even know?

Just as in the outpatient realm, tailoring the patient's discharge instructions to his ability to understand and carry them out is important to implementation and to keeping the patient from being quickly readmitted to the hospital. Yet according to at least one study, the majority of patients interviewed following discharge from the hospital described this aspect of physician-patient communication as being the most lacking.[36]

To see whether physicians were aware of the extent to which patients do not understand their discharge instructions, one group of researchers interviewed eighty-three patients who had all recently gone home after having been admitted to a large teaching hospital for either pneumonia or a heart attack. They also interviewed the attending physicians who had overseen these specific patients' care during their hospitalization. The patients and the physicians were asked about the predischarge instructions that had been given to the patients by their physicians and about the patients' understanding of these instructions.

The findings were remarkable. Although 89 percent of the physicians were certain that their patients had fully comprehended the potential side effects of the medications they were being sent home on, only 57 percent of patients felt the same. Likewise, whereas almost 95 percent of physicians felt that their patients understood when they might be able to return to their normal activities, only 58 percent of the patients agreed.[37] In other words, the physicians assumed that their patients understood these two critical determinants of medical adherence at least 50 percent more than they, the patients, actually did. This misperception of patient comprehension by physicians is alarming, and, as bad as they sound, these findings likely underrepresent the true scope of the problem because they do not account for those patients who believed that they understood what they had been told but in fact did not.

Half of the Medicare patients who wind up readmitted to the hospital within thirty days of discharge turn out not to have been seen by their own primary-care physician during the period between discharge and readmission.[38] It is highly likely that scheduling routine posthospitalization follow-up visits with patients' primary-care physicians would reduce both readmission rates and emergency room visits (more than 7 percent of patients discharged from the hospital are treated in an emergency room within thirty days of discharge).[39] At these visits, the new treatment plans could be reviewed, reinforced, or modified by the patients' regular physician, with whom longstanding relationships and trust are much more likely to exist. The possible side effects of medications and their potential for interaction with others that the patient was already taking could be discussed, reassurances given, and substitutions made if the ones prescribed upon discharge prove to be intolerable or ineffective. This might be the case, for example, if the bacteria that had caused the patient's urinary tract infection turned out not to be sensitive to the oral antibiotics prescribed or if the patient's blood pressure had now become dangerously low because of one of the new heart medications that was started during the most recent admission.

BETTER PHYSICIAN-PATIENT COMMUNICATION INCREASES THE USE OF PREVENTIVE MEDICAL SERVICES

Better communication between patients and physicians leads to the better use of preventive medical services such as cancer screening, for example.[40] When done thoughtfully, preventive care not only results in better health in many instances but is also cost effective.

From a pediatrician's perspective, nothing better exemplifies preventive medicine than vaccines, which have proven to be one of the greatest accomplishments of Western biomedicine. Vaccines save millions of lives annually and enabled the eradication of smallpox in 1979. Yet despite this simple truth, growing numbers of parents do not immunize their children as recommended. A recent study published in *Pediatrics* found that 13 percent of American parents of young children were not vaccinating their children according to the routine schedule. Nine percent of the parents surveyed had refused some or all of the regular childhood immunizations for their children.[41]

Not being vaccinated doesn't just place the specific child at risk of infection with an utterly preventable and potentially deadly disease. It also endangers others with whom they come in contact, especially those with compromised or deficient immune systems who are unable to mount an adequate defense against infection, even if they've already been vaccinated. These include the very young and the very old, solid-organ and bone-marrow transplant recipients, people with AIDS, and those being treated for cancer or autoimmune diseases. Such people, and there are millions of them in the United States alone, rely on *herd immunity* for their protection. This is a concept that refers to the percentage of a given population that needs to be immune to a specific infectious disease in order to prevent an isolated incidence of infection from spreading widely and triggering an epidemic. The herd-immunity threshold varies among diseases depending upon their virulence. To prevent a widespread outbreak of measles, for example, between 92 and 94 percent of the population needs to be immune.[42]

Unfortunately, the rise in the number of parents choosing not to vaccinate their children in recent years is something that anyone working in pediatrics can attest to. More often than I ever would have thought possible, I meet parents who have refused some or all immunization for their children. When asked why, they invariably provide well-thought-out answers. For most, the decision not to vaccinate their children is not the product of laziness or indifference. There is no question that these parents love their kids just as much as any other parent. If anything, they often seem to have done more research on the topic than have many of the parents who adhere to the recommended vaccination schedule.

The reasons that some parents give for not vaccinating their children include any and all of the following: wanting to let their child's immune system function "naturally" without artificial intervention, a reluctance to subject their child to something they aren't convinced is absolutely necessary, and concern that the multiple shots involved will inflict too much discomfort and pain. In addition to these reasons, and often right at the top of the list, is a fear that the vaccines may adversely affect their child's development and behavior.

Ever since the British physician Andrew Wakefield's notorious—and now thoroughly discredited—paper was published in 1998 linking the MMR (measles, mumps, rubella) vaccine with autism, a widespread belief connecting the two stubbornly persists. This remains so even though the paper has since been retracted and Wakefield barred from practicing medicine in the United Kingdom.[43] Largely as a result of the publicity surrounding the controversy, annual MMR vaccination rates in Britain plummeted from 90 percent and greater before Wakefield's article to 79 percent in 2003. The consequences were not long in following. Because of the reduction in personal and herd immunity, the United Kingdom saw a dramatic increase in the annual number of measles cases, with at least fourteen deaths attributed to it between the years 1998 and 2008.[44]

In a recent large study by the Centers for Disease Control and Prevention (CDC) that surveyed parents of young children, more than one-quarter reported concerns that vaccines can cause "learning disabilities such as autism." Eighty-one percent of the parents described their child's doctor or nurse as an important source of information in helping them reach their decision to vaccinate their kids. Significantly, this last number corresponds almost perfectly to the percentage of parents who described themselves as "confident" or "very confident" about the safety and importance of vaccines to their child's health.[45] However, many of the other information sources that the parents described as important in shaping their decisions about vaccinations—family (47 percent), friends (23 percent), various media outlets (10.9 percent), and the Internet (9.9 percent)—have the propensity to provide partial, skewed, and even blatantly false information. The first page of a Google search for "MMR vaccine autism" at the time of this writing, for example, included a link to a recent court case in Italy in which damages were awarded to the family of a fifteen-month-old boy. In that case, the Italian court ruled that the child had become autistic after being given the MMR vaccine, despite extensive expert medical testimony to the contrary.[46]

Returning to the CDC study, it is worth asking why more than 18 percent of those parents surveyed discounted their pediatricians' recommendations about vaccinations for their children. That they did reveals a serious communication gap between them and their children's pediatricians. It also exposes broader weaknesses within the very health care–provision frameworks ostensibly designed to nurture and support that relationship. Unsure of what to do and whom to listen to, these parents sought answers to their health questions elsewhere or chose simply to rely on their gut feelings without engaging the very person—their child's pediatrician—whom one would expect to be the best source for science-based guidance specifically tailored to their values and cultural sensitivities.

"Oh yes, I remember *that* conversation," the mother of a previously unvaccinated three-year-old told me recently at a follow-up visit. I had just asked her if she ever did take her daughter to the pediatrician for the shots she had so steadfastly refused, following my urging her to do so six months earlier when we first met. At that previous visit, I had taken time away from discussing the child's asthma—the reason she had been referred to me in the first place—to try to understand better why her parents had chosen not to vaccinate her and to explain why I felt it was important that she be immunized. At that visit, both mother and father had spoken passionately and at length about their fears that the vaccinations might further hinder their daughter's development, already noticeably delayed and an issue of great concern to them both. Reflecting on that visit afterward, I worried that I might have come down on them too harshly and expected that I might never again see them as a result. But here they were again, back in my office.

Gazing down at her daughter, whose head was resting in her lap, the girl's mother gently brushed some stray wisps of hair away from her face, paused, and said: "She's already gotten three since we saw you last spring. We've decided to space them out, but it's going OK so far."

And then, looking back up at me: "Thank you."

BETTER COMMUNICATION BETWEEN PHYSICIANS AND PATIENTS SAVES MONEY

Better communication between physicians and patients reduces the incidence of adverse events within the hospital setting, such as wrong-side surgery and medication errors, which can result in lengthier and more complicated stays. Not surprisingly, hospitalized patients whose ability to communicate is impeded by language barriers, deafness, or blindness are three times more likely to experience adverse events than the general population.[47]

In the outpatient setting, better communication between patients and physicians leads to more judicious use of medical resources, which in turn reduces costs. One study found that utilizing a model of patient-centered communication led to an 11 percent reduction in the ordering of diagnostic testing and a 3.2 percent reduction in overall expenditures even when increased visit length was taken into account.[48] Why was this so? Probably because more diagnoses were being made through careful history taking and physical examination, necessitating fewer expensive tests. In addition, because their physicians spent more time with them, it is likely that the patients were more inclined to believe their physicians when told, for example, that they really didn't need that spinal MRI to work up their lower-back pain.

When a patient presents with new-onset lower-back pain, it's much easier—and quicker in the short term—for the physician to order an MRI than it is to take a detailed history, perform a thorough physical examination, and provide reassurance based upon experience. However, an MRI also entails a lot of running around for the patient, in most cases provides no added benefit to either patient or physician, and is more costly to the system as a whole. This is why the American College of Physicians now recommends that physicians not order them routinely.[49] In addition, there is also the risk of significant discomfort to the patient if incidental abnormalities that are discovered require further testing and evaluation, which also incurs added expense. The savings that could be realized by avoiding unnecessary imaging studies in patients with lower-back pain have been calculated to be in excess of $300 million annually.[50]

The connection between more face time between patients and physicians leading to less testing and lower overall costs is one worth pondering. Many physicians assume that patients generally want more tests, more medicine, and more care, and, indeed, there is some evidence to bear this out.[51] However, just because some physicians reinforce the misconception that more is better doesn't mean that it's true or even that the physicians themselves believe it to be so. One study, in which more than six hundred primary-care physicians were asked about their attitudes toward the care their patients received, found that 42 percent of the physicians felt that their *own* patients were overtreated. Forty percent felt that not having enough time to spend with their patients led them to adopt a more aggressive style of practice that relied on more testing than on history taking or examination.[52] This would seem to indicate that cutting back on physician face time with patients in the name of so-called efficiency winds up being less efficient for a variety of reasons, as well as less satisfying to all involved.

BETTER COMMUNICATION IS ALSO BETTER FOR PHYSICIANS

Physicians are 36 percent more likely than the general population of working adults to exhibit at least one sign of burnout. Indeed, physician dissatisfaction with how medicine is practiced is widespread, with almost half reporting that they would choose a different profession were they to start their careers anew and only 32 percent willing to recommend medicine as a career to their own children.[53]

Physician burnout is associated with decreased patient satisfaction and with worse clinical outcomes. This explains why poor physician-patient communication has repeatedly been found to result in more complaints to medical regulatory authorities and in more malpractice suits against physicians. This, in turn, increases malpractice insurance premiums, which are rolled into charges for medical services. In addition to the direct costs of defending a malpractice lawsuit, which can be significant, there are also the indirect costs. The average physician spends more than four years disputing an unresolved malpractice claim. This consumes valuable time that would otherwise be spent seeing patients and furthering the physician's education and reduces productivity because of the emotional drain associated with the whole process.[54]

Job dissatisfaction and burnout also lead to physician attrition, which is costly to the health-care system and society. It has been calculated that the cost of recruiting a replacement physician ranges anywhere between $97,000 and $1 million, depending upon the level of the physician and the framework to which he or she is being recruited.[55]

CLOSING THOUGHTS

In this chapter, I've discussed the strong effect that good communication has on improving diagnosis and adherence as well as on reducing costs within the health-care system. These are powerful arguments in favor of paying close attention to the ways in which the different cost-cutting measures currently being proposed and implemented affect this fundamental aspect of health-care provision. Although hard to quantify and tally on a spreadsheet, the net result of better communication between patients and physicians is increased value, defined as outcomes divided by cost, and it is critical not to lose sight of this.

In the next chapter, I'll discuss how better communication between physician and patient enables patient care to be more personalized, making it more likely to succeed, and I will explore the powerful intrinsic therapeutic properties of the physician-patient relationship itself.

2

ONE SIZE DOES *NOT* FIT ALL

Every human benefit, every virtue and every prudent act,
is founded on compromise.

—Edmund Burke

THE PARENTS of a seven-year-old child named Isabelle brought her to see me for a third opinion about how best to manage her obstructive sleep apnea (OSA). This is a condition in which the muscles of the throat collapse during sleep, blocking the flow of air into the lungs and preventing normal breathing. This leads to repeated choking and gasping for air that interrupt the child's sleep. It also causes repeated drops in blood-oxygen levels, which, when severe, can cause injury to the brain, heart, and other organs.

Isabelle and her parents had traveled quite a distance to see me that afternoon, and the first thing I noticed as I entered the clinic room was how nervous Isabelle's parents appeared to be. Something, especially about the mother, seemed different from most parents whom I meet for the first time, in a way that was hard for me to put my finger on. Perhaps it was her weak handshake or the relatively little eye contact she made with me, even though she was the one who did almost all of the talking during that visit, her husband staying mostly silent. Whatever it was, I felt that something was definitely off about her manner.

Isabelle had been born three months prematurely, which had resulted in a host of complications, including a severe brain bleed that had left her profoundly developmentally delayed and quadriplegic. She was nonverbal and noninteractive, was blind, had seizures several times an hour despite the multiple antiseizure medications she was on, and received all of her nutrition and fluids through a feeding tube implanted in her stomach. She was also on supplemental oxygen around the clock.

Because she snored loudly, Isabelle had been referred some months earlier for a sleep study, which was when she had been diagnosed with OSA. I was not surprised at this: although she was awake and sitting upright in her chair when I saw her that afternoon, her breathing was still much noisier than normal. I thought that her OSA was probably caused by a number of factors. She had low muscle tone, which meant that all of her muscles, including those of her tongue and throat, were more relaxed at baseline than most children's. Her head was disproportionately small, something which is often seen in children who have sustained extensive brain damage as infants. This leaves less room for the tongue inside the mouth, forcing it back into the throat, where it can block the normal flow of air into the lungs. Her jaw, too, was unusually shaped. It was very small and set back in her face, leaving her with a severe underbite that kept her mouth fixed open about half an inch, causing her to drool incessantly.

After the sleep study, Isabelle had been seen by two other pediatric pulmonologists. Both had independently told her parents that she needed a tracheostomy. Also called a *trache* (rhymes with rake), a tracheostomy is a short breathing tube inserted directly into the windpipe through a small hole in the front of the throat, which secures the airway and prevents its obstruction. Not pleased with this, they had come to see me to find out whether other options might be available.

I suggested that we try the use of continuous positive airway pressure (CPAP), given by a machine that blows air into the throat via a mask worn over the nose and/or mouth. The pressurized air props the throat open and prevents its collapse. Although they had heard of CPAP before and were very skeptical about whether Isabelle would be able to tolerate its use, after a long discussion they agreed to try it, and I arranged for her to come into the sleep lab so that we could determine what the optimal pressure settings would be for her.

Unfortunately, Isabelle's parents were right. Because of the unusual shape of her head and the fact that she breathed through an open mouth, none of the CPAP masks we had fit properly. Despite their best efforts, the techs were unable to find appropriate CPAP settings to successfully overcome her OSA.

A few days later, Isabelle's parents and I met again. Not surprisingly, they were even more discouraged than before.

"So I guess this means that there's no choice, and Isabelle needs a trache?" her mother asked glumly, briefly meeting my eyes before turning toward her daughter to wipe a trickle of saliva from her chin with a corner of an already sodden bandana.

This was when I started to grasp what the real reason was for them having come to see me in the first place.

I told them that I thought that there were, in fact, at least three options available for Isabelle. One possibility was a trache, and while I explained how this might help their daughter, I also pointed out that traches, too, have complications, such as getting plugged with mucus and secretions, becoming infected, and triggering bleeds that in some cases can be fatal. Isabelle's parents were well aware of all of this. They were members of a support group for parents of children with profound developmental delay, many of whom were trached.

Another treatment option, I continued, might be for Isabelle to have reconstructive craniofacial surgery to rebuild her face and jaw so that she would have more room to breathe. I also explained, however, that this might not succeed in curing her OSA and that the process itself would be a long one, likely involving multiple surgeries and associated with significant discomfort at every step. Watching the shift in their body language, I could see that this appealed to them even less than a trache did.

Finally, I told them that I thought that it was also entirely reasonable to do nothing more than they were currently doing for her, that is, continuing to give her supplemental oxygen at night to blunt the drops in her blood-oxygen levels. While it is certainly true that untreated OSA can cause cognitive impairment in some children, this was not, unfortunately, a real concern in Isabelle, who was already neurologically devastated. And although having untreated obstructive sleep apnea would put her at increased risk of heart disease and other medical problems, these could be somewhat mitigated by keeping her blood-oxygen levels within a normal range with the supplemental oxygen. As it was, I continued, we needed to remember that Isabelle was already a high-risk child because of her many other medical problems and that this would not change, regardless of how aggressively we decided to treat her OSA.

I concluded by emphasizing to Isabelle's parents that I felt that any of these treatment options would be acceptable. I suggested that they take some time to decide on the balance they wished to strike between aggressive intervention and keeping her comfortable, based upon what they felt was most appropriate for her.

Isabelle's parents were silent for about twenty seconds as they processed what I had just told them. And then, abruptly, her mother leaned forward and looked me straight in the eye.

"So are you saying that Isabelle *doesn't* need a trache?"

"No," I answered. "What I'm saying is that you have choices and that I'll support you in whatever decision you make."

This was a pivotal moment. Isabelle's mother proceeded to open up to me as she hadn't ever before. She explained that both she and Isabelle's father felt that it was of utmost importance that Isabelle be comfortable. Above all, she said, they wanted to avoid any interventions that might cause her to suffer or that would adversely affect the quality of her life, even if the result would be that her life would be shorter. Following a recent hospitalization for pneumonia a couple months earlier, her parents had discussed whether they would even want to bring her to the hospital the next time she became sick. After witnessing how miserable Isabelle had seemed while intubated and mechanically ventilated, they felt that it would be better for her if they could just care for her at home. There, they would be able to hydrate her and give her feeds and antibiotics through the feeding tube, as well as continue to give her the oxygen she was already on.

"We already have a mini-hospital set up at home," said Isabelle's mother.

"What we really *don't* want, though, is for her to have to undergo aggressive resuscitation or to have to have an autopsy if she dies at home," said her father, speaking up for the first time that day.

The longer we spoke, the more I knew that my hunch about why they had come to see me in the first place was correct. Although they believed it unlikely, Isabelle's parents had hoped that I would be able to offer a less aggressive, and in their opinion more appropriate, treatment course for their daughter. They had felt they were being coerced into doing something to Isabelle that they disagreed with, by a medical system that didn't seem to place any value on what they as her parents thought best for her.

Isabelle's parents may have been as reserved with her other physicians as they initially were with me about what they wanted the parameters of her care to be, at least until I raised the possibility of treating her less aggressively, describing that option as being just as legitimate as any of the others. It's hard to blame them, though. Many parents of medically complex children in this position have difficulty overcoming the guilt they feel at being bad parents for not wanting to do everything possible for their child. This is especially true when the parents somehow blame themselves for their child's condition. *If only I had been more careful, perhaps I wouldn't have gone into preterm labor, and then she wouldn't have bled into her brain the way she did.* This becomes even harder to overcome when their child's physicians express clear preferences for a more aggressive approach at odds with what the parents, in their hearts, feel would be best for their child. Isabelle's parents really, *really* did not want her to be trached, as I learned, but felt that they were being pressured into agreeing to one by their daughter's physicians.

I contacted one of our social workers, and we connected the family with the hospital's Pediatric Advanced Care Team. Together we arranged for Isabelle to be designated as a comfort-care recipient. This would allow her to be cared for in her home if she were to get sick and even to die there peacefully, if and when it came to that, without having to undergo either resuscitation or autopsy.

I didn't see Isabelle for more than four years after that and had almost forgotten about her, until one day her parents brought her to in to see me again in the clinic. Isabelle was in pretty much the same condition, apart from a worsening of her scoliosis. An orthopedist had recommended doing spinal surgery to correct the curvature of her back, which was contorting her chest and constricting her lungs. In anticipation of the surgery, the orthopedist had suggested placing a trache so that Isabelle's airway could be optimally managed.

Isabelle's parents' views on how best to manage her care hadn't changed since I'd last seen her. If anything, they'd strengthened and become more well defined. Her parents were very forthcoming this time about why they had come back to see me. They really were not interested in the back surgery at all, given its risks and the inevitable discomfort it would cause Isabelle. The question of whether she should be trached in advance of the surgery was merely an excuse for the visit. What they really wanted, they readily told me, was reassurance that it would be OK if they chose not to proceed with the back surgery, even if the result would be that her lungs would be progressively compressed as her chest slowly collapsed.

Once again I reiterated to them that I thought that they were excellent parents; that this, too, was a complicated choice between two uncertain and imperfect outcomes; and that both choices seemed reasonable to me. They left satisfied and, as far as I know, have decided not to go ahead with the back surgery.

I've shared this story to show that while most patients come to physicians in straightforward search of treatment, there are also those, such as Isabelle's parents, whose agenda may be atypical and quite different from what is initially presented. Although Isabelle's parents struggled with what they perceived as a natural inclination of the medical system to be overly aggressive with her care, they had little choice but to rely upon it. The two specialists who had seen Isabelle before me had very appropriately described to her parents what *could* be done for her but had not engaged them in the equally important conversation about what *should* be done for her.

While many physicians and parents might have chosen to treat Isabelle differently, I would disagree with those who might argue that her parents' decisions, which I supported, were somehow unethical. Choosing among a trache, craniofacial surgery, back surgery, or supportive care meant selecting one of many possibilities, each of which entailed risks and offered benefits the others did not. This is why there was no right answer, certainly not from an ethical perspective.

As David Browning, MSW, a cofounder of the Institute for Professionalism and Ethical Practice at Boston Children's Hospital, has pointed out: "The only reason that such difficult choices exist in the first place is because of technological advances which have outpaced our ability, as a society, to know how best to help families decide whether and when to take advantage of them."[1] The very existence of diverse and strongly held opinions about what to do in situations such as these is a testament to it remaining a highly charged and still unresolved issue.

DECISIONS ON INTENSITY OF TREATMENT AND END-OF-LIFE CARE

It is fascinating to realize that many physicians do not practice what they preach, at least regarding the aggressiveness of the care they would choose for themselves versus what they recommend to their own patients. This is borne out by the findings of a large study of primary-care physicians who were asked what treatment they would choose for themselves were they to be hypothetically diagnosed with colon cancer, versus what treatment they would recommend for a patient of theirs with a similar diagnosis. The choice was between a conservative treatment regimen with fewer side effects and a lower chance of survival and a more aggressive treatment regimen with more side effects and a higher chance of survival. Almost 38 percent of the physicians chose the more conservative treatment for themselves, compared to only 25 percent who said that they would have recommended it to a patient of theirs.[2]

This tendency of physicians to be more conservative with their own medical care was eloquently described by Ken Murray, a clinical assistant professor of family medicine at the University of Southern California, in two articles he wrote for *Zócalo Public Square*: "How Doctors Die" and "Doctors Really Do Die Differently." Murray told the story of a dying patient of his and of how he had helped the patient's family reach a decision about redirecting care goals from aggressive intervention to provision of comfort. After describing some of the possible reasons why physicians might "do everything they can" even in cases with virtually no hope of recovery, such as avoiding lawsuits or possible prosecution for homicide or for financial reasons, he wrote: "It's no wonder many doctors err on the side of overtreatment. But doctors still don't over-treat themselves. They see the consequences of this constantly. Almost anyone can find a way to die in peace at home, and pain can be managed better than ever."[3]

Laypeople, unfortunately, do not have anywhere near the same kind of familiarity with what end-of-life care looks like. Unless they discuss it with their physicians, both patients and their families have very limited ability to make informed decisions about how they would like their own end-of-life care to be administered. The absence of a decision is in itself a decision of sorts, with the default usually being to push on with painful and unpleasant treatments that only serve to delay the inevitable and that are excruciating for the patient's loved ones to witness. These treatments are also very costly, despite their poor yield. The *Wall Street Journal* recently reported that 22.3 percent of the total Medicare expenditures on hospital care in 2009 were generated by the 6.6 percent of patients who died that year, more than $172 billion.[4] Unfortunately, had they been asked, in many cases the patients themselves would have requested that less aggressive measures be taken to extend their lives, not because of the monetary costs but because of the physical and mental suffering they inevitably cause.

The vast majority of Americans do, in fact, express a desire for advance end-of-life care planning.[5] Recognizing this, a provision to reimburse physicians for voluntarily counseling Medicare patients about end-of-life issues such as hospice care and living wills was originally introduced as part of the Patient Protection and Affordable Care Act (Obamacare). However, following its demonization as paving the way for the establishment of "death panels," this provision was withdrawn.[6]

This is unfortunate: advance-care directives created by patients after discussing their end-of-life choices and preferences with their physicians and loved ones enable those who suffer from chronic or terminal disease to make rational and well-thought-out choices about their care. These directives reflect the patients' own personal outlooks and preferences and allow them to live—and to die—with dignity. The directives can also be expanded to include advance planning for the care patients might want to receive in the event of an unanticipated catastrophe such as a massive stroke or motor vehicle accident, which leaves them in a persistent vegetative state.

During the discussions that lead up to the creation of these directives, the patient learns about what can and cannot be done in specific circumstances and what the implications of various treatment options would be from the perspectives of pain, function, and overall quality of life. Conversations about end-of-life care decrease the use of aggressive treatments in the last thirty days of life, including hospitalization, intensive care–unit stays, and chemotherapy, while at the same time increasing hospice-care utilization.[7] All of these save considerable expense to the health-care system and society by preventing situations in which physicians are directed by family members to "do everything" they can to save Grandpa, regardless of the consequences. All too often, this doing everything means performing heroic procedures that offer only a very small chance of success while at the same time causing significant discomfort and merely prolonging the dying process. Had Grandpa himself been consulted, he might well have asked that things be done altogether differently.

Much remains to be improved upon in this area. One large study known by its acronym as the SUPPORT study (Study to Understand Prognoses and Preferences for Outcomes and Risks of Treatments) was conducted to research end-of-life preferences and improve the end-of-life care of seriously ill patients. The SUPPORT study enrolled more than nine thousand patients diagnosed with one of nine life-threatening conditions and found that by the third day of their hospitalization only 23 percent had discussed their resuscitation preferences with their physicians. Forty-two percent of those who had not done so expressed regret about this.[8] Clearly, both physicians and patients need to be more proactive about discussing advance-care planning, preferably even before the issues arise and the patient, his family, and physician are all faced with making difficult decisions in moments of extreme stress. It allows for a deliberate, well-thought-out, and agreed-upon set of directives to be developed in advance and then implemented in real time, preventing needless suffering and reducing unnecessary expense.

NEGOTIATION BETWEEN PHYSICIAN AND PATIENT

One of the most important insights that I gained while learning how to care for patients with cystic fibrosis (CF) during the first year of my pediatric pulmonary fellowship was the importance of negotiation between physician and patient over the parameters and goals of treatment. Without buy-in from the patient, I learned, the likelihood of any treatment succeeding diminishes, regardless of how authoritative or knowledgeable the physician is—or thinks he is.

The process of negotiation between physician and patient allows the patient to mold what the physician proposes into something that conforms to her own belief system and values. It also forces the physician to acknowledge and address ahead of time concerns that the patient may have and that might otherwise pose significant hurdles to adherence. The process of negotiation, too, is often an important milestone on the patient's path of adjustment to, and acceptance of, life with chronic disease. This corresponds to the stage of bargaining, the third of the five stages of grief described by the psychiatrist Elisabeth Kübler-Ross in her classic book *On Death and Dying.*[9] By promoting and encouraging this process, the physician becomes not merely a physical healer but a spiritual one as well.

I was almost four months into my fellowship when I went up to the tenth floor of the hospital one late October afternoon to admit a new patient to the pulmonary service. Jamie, a young woman in her early twenties, had been admitted because of a worsening of her cystic-fibrosis-related lung disease, which necessitated intravenous antibiotic treatment, supplemental oxygen, and intense chest physical therapy.

CF is the most common genetic disease in Caucasians. It affects approximately one in 2,500 pregnancies and is caused by genetic mutations that impair the ability of cells to transport chloride across their outer walls. This leads to the production and accumulation of very thick and sticky secretions in the lungs (and other organs) that are difficult to dislodge and expel. The secretions become chronically infected, damaging and scarring the lungs and leading to their progressive loss of function. It is this steady loss of lung function that ultimately causes the early death of most patients with CF. Currently, the median life expectancy for people with this disease is around thirty-eight. At some point, the work of breathing becomes too great for these patients' damaged lungs to sustain. This can happen abruptly because of an acute respiratory infection that suddenly overwhelms them, or it can occur at the end of a slow and steady decline, when the lungs become so scarred that they are simply no longer able to transport oxygen and carbon dioxide in and out of the bloodstream effectively.

Regardless of how quickly or slowly the decline in lung function occurs, the goals of the physician and the patient are to try to prevent it from happening altogether or, at the very least, to delay its progression as much as possible. This is attempted with a variety of treatments, some preventive, and others that are given to the patient while acutely ill. At present, there is no cure for CF, and although lung transplantation presents an opportunity for some patients with advanced disease, that, too, has risks and complications. This is why maintaining lung function and preventing its decline in these patients is so important.

Entering the room, I said hello to Jamie, who was sitting on the bed with her legs crossed in front of her. Before coming upstairs to see her, I had reviewed her chart and chest X rays and had already thought about which antibiotics might be the most appropriate to treat her with. As I sat across from her, Jamie told me about the increasing shortness of breath she'd been experiencing over the previous two weeks. This had been accompanied by an increase in her cough and sputum production. She told me that she was now bringing up mouthfuls of thick, mostly dark-green mucous—she had collected perhaps four ounces in the cup by her bedside during the two hours since she'd arrived—that had been blood-tinged the night before, "but not today," she hastened to reassure me. Jamie's appetite had also gone down significantly, and she now weighed several pounds less than she had one month earlier, an ominous sign.

Running through my mental checklists, I asked Jamie about problems in other organ systems, those commonly affected by CF as well as others not usually involved. I reviewed her medication list, asked about allergies, and was almost done with the interview when I asked, almost off-handedly, whether she had had any recent exposure to other sick people, animals, mold, or cigarette smoke.

"Cigarettes? No way," she responded vehemently. "I don't go anywhere near people who smoke cigarettes. Those are really bad for me." Satisfied, I began to stand up so that I could examine her. Jamie continued, "I only smoke the three cigars a week that Dr. Wohl said I could, and that's it. Otherwise, I don't go anywhere near tobacco."

Taken completely off guard, I sat right back down again and looked at her closely, trying to read her. Though at first I thought that she was joking, something about Jamie's expression was convincing. She then told me that her grandfather had smoked cigars when she was younger and that she had always loved the smell. She herself had begun smoking cigars soon after turning fifteen.

"You understand, don't you, that cigars are just as bad for your lungs as cigarettes, maybe even worse, because they don't have filters?" I asked, still not entirely sure of whether or not she was pulling my leg.

Jamie paused, squinted at me slightly, and then reminded me—as if I needed reminding—that her primary pulmonologist happened to be my division chief, a woman of international reputation with more years of experience treating patients with CF than I had been alive for.

"If Dr. Wohl says it's OK for me to smoke three cigars a week, that's good enough for me," she said. She continued to stare at me for a couple more seconds, and then looked away.

It was obvious that Jamie was done discussing this issue. The rest of the visit was a bit awkward. I proceeded with her examination, reviewed the treatment plan with her, and bid her farewell for the day.

As luck would have it, on the way back to my office I ran into Dr. Wohl, who too was just coming back from seeing another patient in clinic. She spotted me and asked how Jamie looked. Sick but stable, I answered, and told her about the care plan I'd come up with. At the end, I repeated to her what Jamie had told me about supposedly having been granted permission to smoke cigars.

Dr. Mary Ellen Beck Wohl, I should point out, was one of the best clinicians I have ever met. She was also a superb teacher and an outstanding mentor. She had a great sense of humor, a huge heart, and a motherly mien toward her faculty, especially her trainees. Dr. Wohl was extremely dedicated and devoted to her patients in ways that were regarded as either legendary or notorious, depending upon whom you asked. I was curious about how she'd respond to what I'd just told her. Would she mock my gullibility, or perhaps take offense at having such a blatant untruth made up about her by one of her patients?

She did neither. Instead, she leaned against the wall, crossed her arms, and cocked her head at me, almost preening. "Pretty ingenious, huh?" she said, smiling.

My bewilderment must have been obvious. She looked down at my hospital ID badge, then back up again at me.

"Jamie doesn't always feel sick, and certainly doesn't want to *be* sick. I can't tell you how much time I've spent struggling to get her to start taking care of herself. The fact that this is the first time in two years that she's needed to be admitted would have seemed nothing short of miraculous five years ago."

"But the cigars . . ." I began.

"She would have smoked them no matter what I told her. However, by 'allowing' her three cigars a week, I empowered her and gave her control over the daily decision making surrounding the management of her own health. I'd be surprised if she smokes more than a dozen a year; she's told me they make her hack for days afterward. But ever since agreeing to take her meds and to do her breathing treatments and chest physical therapy in exchange for those three weekly cigars, she's done so, so much better."

I was astonished, though in hindsight I shouldn't have been. This was the same Dr. Wohl who sometimes paid kids in cash to take their medicines. The same Dr. Wohl who would ask her younger patients to stand up on their beds during rounds so that she could examine their lungs because "most kids get yelled at when they stand on the bed, so this is how I let them get away with secretly breaking the rules."

Many of the other physicians in the division, myself included, disagreed with how Dr. Wohl bribed some of her more stubbornly nonadherent patients to carry out their treatments. It seemed to transform the treatments from something the patients needed to do for *themselves* into something they did for *her.* But by negotiating Jamie's adherence in exchange for permission to smoke a certain number of cigars at her discretion, what Dr. Wohl was actually doing was giving Jamie a measure of autonomy and even some limited mastery over what is truly an oppressive and relentless disease. Jamie no longer felt totally adrift and at the mercy of whatever CF and her physicians threw at her. Instead, for the first time in her life, Jamie had been given the opportunity to make choices about her own care rather than meekly submitting to what she was told she needed to do. Enjoying the occasional cigar also allowed Jamie to detach herself from the sick role that CF had thrust upon her, even if only for brief periods of time (I'll return to how the sick role as defined by society becomes central to many patients' self-identity, especially those suffering from chronic disease, in chapter 4). The resulting better health outcomes and higher self-esteem for Jamie were precisely in line with what Dr. Wohl wanted for her and for all of her other patients, and they satisfied both immensely. The fact that these were achieved through unorthodox means hardly mattered and seems entirely beside the point.

PLACEBOS AND THE IMPORTANCE OF PATIENT BELIEF AND HOPE

Empowering patients to take control and mastery of their disease is but one of the many ways in which the interaction between physician and patient directly influences outcomes. The encouragement and reassurance conveyed by the physician are no less important in helping the patient enlist the inner strength necessary to fight his disease and not despair.

One of the more interesting phenomena in medicine is the response elicited by placebos, Latin for "I shall please," mediated directly by the communication between physician and patient. Placebos are nonactive substances that are sometimes given by a physician to his patient to placate her complaints when he has no other good solutions to offer. In these cases, placebos are usually given under the guise of being an actual medication with therapeutic properties. When used to treat pain, for example, the success rates of placebos can vary considerably. Many studies show that placebos can reduce pain in large numbers of patients who receive them, greater even than the 35 percent rate first reported by Henry Beecher in 1955.[10] Placebos are also often given as part of clinical trials evaluating the relative efficacy of a study drug, in order to assess the drug's effect while canceling out the effect that just being given *something*, believed to be beneficial by the person receiving it, may have.

How, precisely, do placebos work? This remains the subject of much debate among scientists. That they do work, however, is not in doubt among most clinicians. One survey of internists affiliated with three Chicago-area medical schools found that 96 percent believed in the therapeutic effects of placebos. Forty-five percent reported having used placebos in their own clinical practice, and only 12 percent felt that doing so should be prohibited as part of routine medical care.[11]

The placebo effect is not restricted to medical treatment alone but extends to surgery as well. Researchers from the University of Denver followed a group of patients with Parkinson's disease who participated in a clinical trial of embryonic stem cell transplantation into the brain to treat their disease. All of the participants underwent a surgical procedure, in which incisions were made in their scalps and holes drilled into their foreheads, while awake and treated only with local anesthesia. At that point, half the participants had embryonic stem cells injected into their brains; the other half did not. None of the participants actually knew for sure whether they had, in fact, received a stem-cell transplant. Half of the patients in each group (treatment and sham) were then told that they had received a stem-cell transplant, meaning that half of those who had not received them thought that they had, and vice versa. Over the subsequent twelve months, the researchers discovered that those who believed that they had received the stem-cell transplant—irrespective of whether or not they actually had—reported a significant improvement in their quality of life relative to those who believed that they hadn't received a transplant.[12]

The placebo effect has both physiological and psychological components. Yet as Plato pointed out more than two millennia ago, attempting to separate the body from the soul very often proves to be a fool's errand. This is especially true when treating pain, which is, after all, an entirely subjective experience. Some investigators have explained the placebo response as a form of conditioning, in which the patient forms expectations about current treatment that are based upon his own previous experiences. Others have found that the mere *expectation* of diminished pain leads to a commensurate reduction in anxiety. This, in turn, results in the priming of so-called reward loops within the brain, causing the release of endorphins and other pain-mitigating neurotransmitters. There is also evidence that at least some of the placebo effect may be mediated by the hormone oxytocin, levels of which can be affected by interpersonal dynamics. One clinical study, for example, found an association between positive interpersonal communication and higher levels of oxytocin and another hormone, vasopressin, which correlated with more rapid wound healing.[13]

The specific mechanisms through which placebos work, however, are ultimately less important than the fact that they do, actually, work. This again underscores how important the interaction between physician and patient is to the healing process, in ways altogether separate from adherence, because of how that specific interaction shapes the patient's expectations of treatment outcomes. Empathy and compassion alone on the part of the physician aren't enough: necessary, too, are hope and belief on the part of the patient that the treatment will successfully treat the disease as intended.

In his book on the physician-patient relationship, *The Doctor, His Patient, and the Illness*, the physician and psychoanalyst Michael Balint wrote that "in spite of our almost pathetic lack of knowledge about the dynamisms and possible consequences of 'reassurance' and 'advice,' these two are perhaps the most often used forms of medical treatment. In other words, they are the most frequent forms in which the drug 'doctor' is administered."[14] Therefore, it is very important that the physician actively promote hope and belief in the treatment being given, whenever realistic. The patient, in turn, acknowledges this by her willingness to carry out the physician's recommendations, which in some instances assume the trappings of ritual: *take this red pill in the morning, precisely half an hour before eating.* The presence of ritual in modern-day biomedicine is consistent with the historic intertwining of the roles of healer and religious authority figure, which persists to this day in many traditional societies, as will be discussed in greater detail in the next chapter.

In Dr. Edward Rosenbaum's memoir *A Taste of My Own Medicine*—later made into the film *The Doctor*—he describes how he learned about the practice of medicine in "the real world" from a more experienced physician during his army service during the Second World War:

> In those days a major infant problem was diarrhea, and there was no specific medical treatment. Davy said his method was: "When the mother consults you, tell her to give the baby chicken soup. Advise her that the soup must be made from a chicken that is exactly eight days old, not seven days, not nine days, but exactly eight-days-old. She will spend a day searching in the markets, and you will avoid frantic calls. By the time she calls you back, the baby will be well."[15]

The treatment itself, whether a recognized pharmaceutical, a traditional remedy (holy water, chicken soup), or a placebo, becomes a vector for the healing intention extended by the healer—in this case, the physician—which the patient then physically internalizes in order to channel its powers into a cure.

Although the placebo effect is extremely significant, it is also very difficult to study from an ethical standpoint. Providing placebos to patients intentionally kept unaware that they are being given a nonactive substance and who instead are led to believe that the "medicine" they are taking has intrinsic healing properties is fraudulent and highly unethical. Regretfully, this has been done far too often in clinical trials conducted by Western pharmaceutical companies in developing countries.[16] This is entirely different, however, from clinical trials in which patients enroll with the clear understanding in advance that there is a 50 percent chance that they *might* be given a placebo.

Still, you might think that once patients become aware that they have been given something possessing absolutely no therapeutic properties, it would become impossible to tease out the placebo effect. This very transparency would seem to defeat the whole purpose of the study by revealing not only its premise but also the very deception necessary for placebos to work their magic. It would be like the scene in *The*

Wizard of Oz in which Toto the dog draws back the drape to reveal that the Wizard is, in fact, just an ordinary person. Once Dorothy and the others see him and disregard his instructions to "pay no attention to that man behind the curtain," his magical powers vanish.

In the case of placebos, however, this is apparently not the case. This was demonstrated recently by a study at Harvard Medical School using *open-label* placebos, meaning that everyone who was given the placebos knew that what they were receiving contained no active ingredients. Eighty adults with irritable-bowel syndrome were recruited for this study, in which half were given what were presented to them as "placebo pills made of an inert substance, like sugar pills, that have been shown in clinical studies to produce significant improvement in irritable-bowel syndrome symptoms through mind-body self-healing processes." The other half were given no treatment whatsoever. All patients spent similar amounts of time with their health-care providers (physicians and nurse practitioners), and the quality of all the study participants' relationships with their health-care providers was described as similar, irrespective of whether or not they were given the placebo.[17]

The results were fascinating. Those patients who had been given placebos reported global improvement in their symptoms, reduced severity of symptoms, and improved quality of life relative to those who had not. The placebo-response rate for this study was very high: 59 percent.[18] Now, it is true that the number of patients enrolled in this study was small and that because it was an open-label study, some of the participants may have told their providers what they thought they wanted to hear. However, these impressive results certainly invite further research and strengthen the notion of the placebo as vector of the healing intention of the physician (and other healers).

The opposite of the placebo is the nocebo, Latin for "I shall harm." The harmful effect of the nocebo can be just as potent as the healing effect of the placebo. In certain cultures, nocebos can cause death, such as in cases when a spell or hex is cast by a figure of authority who is usually believed also to possess healing powers. In our society, the nocebo effect has been documented in patients who have been warned about the possible side effects of certain medications. Those to whom these side effects were exaggerated prior to starting the medication reported experiencing them more frequently than others to whom the same side effects were downplayed.[19]

Another example of the nocebo effect was demonstrated by a study done on a group of women in labor receiving either epidural or spinal anesthesia. Women who were told prior to the procedure that it was going to be very uncomfortable reported experiencing significantly more pain than those to whom the procedure was described in much more gentle terms. Nocebos affect not just subjective measures of pain and anxiety, but also cause objective physiologic changes, such as increased levels of blood cortisol, a stress hormone.[20] The centrality of physician-patient communication in eliciting the nocebo effect, clearly undesirable, mirrors its role with the placebo effect and underscores its intrinsic importance to the healing process.

CLOSING THOUGHTS

In this chapter, I've discussed the importance of good communication between physician and patient in helping the patient choose and negotiate treatments and desired health outcomes consistent with his wishes and core values. I've also explored some of the intrinsic healing properties of Balint's "drug doctor," administered directly by the physician to the patient. This is a potent medicine that physicians—especially at the beginning of their careers—can easily overlook while concentrating on the more technical aspects of disease treatment, to the exclusion of the patient's many other needs. Key to its delivery is the active communication, by the physician to the patient, of the respect and compassion she has for him.

In the next chapter, I'll explore some of the ways that cultural differences between patient and physician, especially those affecting disease conceptualization, can complicate this communication tremendously.

3

WHEN WORLDS COLLIDE

Homo sum, humani nihil a me alienum puto
[I am human, nothing human is alien to me].

—Terence, Roman playwright (195–159 BCE)

DURING MY pediatrics residency in Israel, much of my on-call time was spent in the pediatric emergency room. The hospital where I trained, Kaplan Medical Center, is located in Rehovot, a small city about half an hour southeast of Tel Aviv. Rehovot is home to the Weizmann Institute of Science and the Faculty of Agriculture of the Hebrew University and has a mixed population of scientists and other academics, career military officers, and mostly middle-class Israelis. Rehovot is also home to a sizable community of Ethiopian Jews, who settled there after immigrating to Israel in the early 1990s.

Much of the ancient Jewish community of Ethiopia, which traces its roots back to the time of the biblical King Solomon and the Queen of Sheba, moved to Israel in two big waves of immigration in the mid 1980s and the early 1990s. While some of the more than seventy thousand immigrants arrived from Addis Ababa and other urban centers, the majority hailed from isolated rural towns located mostly in Gondar province, and their absorption was much more difficult than that of other immigrant groups to Israel. When comparing how the Ethiopian Jews fared relative to the more than one million immigrants who arrived in Israel from the former Soviet Union during the same period, for example, one sees that the Ethiopians as a group, especially those who were older than thirty upon their arrival, had a much harder time finding employment and assimilating into the larger Israeli society. Some of this had to do with learning a new language and adapting to different ways of doing things, but these difficulties were compounded by the immigrants having to adjust to a modern industrial society radically different from the one they had left behind. This ranged from simple things, such as learning about indoor plumbing, to some of the more complex aspects of everyday life in Israel. The new immigrants needed to learn how to use credit cards and checking accounts, how to receive the government assistance they were entitled to, and how to navigate a modern health-care system for themselves and their families.

In addition to these hardships, many of the dark-skinned Ethiopian immigrants encountered racism, sometimes overt, other times disguised as pseudoreligious concerns. Because many of the immigrants, especially the older ones, lacked marketable skills, it was difficult for them to find all but the most menial work and to make the personal connections with other Israelis that could have helped them break down the cultural barriers and walls of discrimination. While this has begun to happen with the next generation, born and educated in Israel, the poor integration of many Ethiopian-born Jews into Israeli society remains one of the failures of a country that, starting out with a population of just six hundred thousand at the time of its founding in 1948, has been remarkably successful in absorbing millions of immigrants from over one hundred countries during its short existence.

It was just after nine p.m. on a hot and sticky Friday night in July 1998 when I met this particular Ethiopian family. The air conditioner in the pediatric emergency room was working full blast but could barely keep the temperature below eighty-five degrees. The air conditioner was half-covered in ice from condensation, and water dripped continuously from its base into a bucket placed underneath. While the frantic pace in the ER had calmed down slightly a couple of hours earlier, while most Israelis were sitting down for the Shabbat (Sabbath) evening meal, it had now picked up again with a vengeance, almost as if everyone were trying to make up for lost time. This was a predictable pattern that played out every Friday night, holiday eve, and whenever there was a big soccer match on television. The only living creatures not scurrying about in that small and crowded pavilion were two small lizards on the ceiling, who seemed to be regarding the hubbub below with detached amusement.

A one-year-old in the small tub in the alcove by the entrance cheerfully splashed his parents with the tepid water, singing and laughing and looking like a totally different child than when he first arrived, now that his fever had broken. In the waiting room, a six-year-old girl was getting a bolus of intravenous (IV) fluids because of dehydration brought on by gastroenteritis; she was still looking pretty beat up. Next to her, a nine-year-old boy with an acute asthma exacerbation sat in his father's lap watching television while his admission forms were being filled out. In the corner, away from everyone else, the parents of a three-day-old infant with neonatal jaundice sat on the edges of their seats, anxiously watching their peacefully sleeping baby. Too nervous to speak, they were waiting to hear if there was an open bed in the neonatal intensive-care unit so that she could be admitted there without having to be exposed to other sick kids in the regular pediatric ward. The four-hundred-square-foot waiting room was filled to capacity. There were perhaps twenty sick children accompanied by at least thirty anxious adults, all wanting their kids to be seen, cured, and sent home quickly so that they, too, could finally get some rest after the long work week.

I picked up the chart of the next kid waiting to be seen and noticed that it belonged to a twenty-day-old girl named Sarah with an Ethiopian surname who had presented with a fever of 102.2. I called out her name and scanned the crowded waiting room as I tried to remember how many open cribs were still available in the ward for new admissions. Fever in a newborn can be caused by many things: dehydration, a viral infection, even overbundling. However, since it can also be the only sign of a serious bacterial infection, febrile babies routinely undergo a full evaluation, including blood, urine, and cerebrospinal fluid cultures, and get admitted for IV antibiotics until the cultures come back sterile. During the first weeks of life, a newborn's immune system is incapable of mounting an effective defense, and if left untreated, bacterial infections at this age can be fatal within hours.

Two people stood up and made their way slowly to the counter. As I had anticipated, they were indeed Ethiopian Jews. The father was a slender man of average height. He had a trimmed goatee and wore a green fedora. He carried a long umbrella, which he used as a walking stick, and had a white shawl draped over one shoulder. Seeing the umbrella, I wondered if they had set out for the hospital on foot that afternoon after public transportation had shut down because of Shabbat and, if so, how long it had taken them to arrive. Taxis were always available, of course, but not everyone could afford them. The umbrella would have been used to shield them from the strong summer sun and had certainly not been brought along because of rain: Israel is dry between April and October. His wife wore a white kerchief on her head as well as a white shawl that covered her back and both shoulders, which she collected in front of herself. An older woman, the grandmother perhaps, remained seated.

The parents followed me into the examination room. Once inside, they continued to stand, the father nervously looking in my general direction and making intermittent eye contact, the mother burying her gaze in the floor. I introduced myself, shook their hands, asked them to be seated, and closed the door behind us. When the mother sat down, she let go of the corners of her shawl, revealing her baby, swaddled and bound tightly to her chest.

The father told me in halting Hebrew that Sarah was their third child and had been born at Kaplan three weeks earlier. There had been no complications with either pregnancy or delivery. Sarah had begun nursing without difficulty and been discharged home with her mother two days later. By the time of her first well-baby visit one week later, Sarah had gained back her birth weight and then some. Everything had been fine until she had started to refuse to nurse the previous day. Her diapers had been dry since early that morning, and she had become increasingly listless and lethargic.

"Did you take her to see a doctor?" I asked, trying to understand if she'd received any treatment earlier that day that might affect what I would need to do for her.

"Yes," replied the father, nodding.

"What did he tell you to do? Did he give you anything for her?" I asked.

Confused, he looked at me and said, "You, you are the doctor." It took me a second before I realized that he meant that this was the first time Sarah had been brought to medical attention since becoming ill.

"Is anybody else sick at home?" I asked.

"No, thank God," he replied. "Everyone at home is healthy, thank God."

I asked the mother if she had anything to add, but the only response I received was a blank stare. The father stated the obvious: she spoke no Hebrew.

I asked them to undress the baby and place her on the examination table. Even before she was fully exposed, I could see that she was in bad shape. She was barely responsive. Her limp extremities were purple and cold, very out of place on such a hot night. Her eyes and fontanel were sunken, and her slightly parted lips exposed pasty-dry gums and tongue. Bending over to examine her, the smell of pus and something rotten coming from her mouth made me shudder.

Inserting a tongue depressor into her mouth, I was appalled by what I saw.

The whole of her soft palate was swollen and dark red, except for that portion where her uvula (the dangling piece of flesh at the back of the throat) should have been. There, a black, dime-size scab partly covered a stump of necrotic tissue that was oozing pus and blood. I knew then what had happened to Sarah. I had already seen other Ethiopian babies who had gone through this as well, but never one as sick as Sarah before. It was now obvious to me why she had fever and was refusing to drink.

"When was this done?" I asked the father, trying to hide my revulsion.

"Two days ago," he answered in a soft, almost passive voice. He looked away from me and from his daughter and wife, almost as if he were trying to will himself somewhere else, anywhere else but this tiny exam room. His shoulders slumped slightly.

Maintaining a neutral tone, I asked him, "Why? Was something the matter? Was she sick?"

He looked back at me, a defeated look on his face, as if acknowledging that escape was impossible.

"No, she was fine, but I was afraid that it would swell up and she would choke on it and die. That's what happened to my brother's son in Gondar, and we didn't want that to happen to her."

"Who did the cutting?" I asked.

"One of the community elders," he replied.

As with all groups of people sharing a common culture and heritage fostered over thousands of years, the Jews of Ethiopia had developed their own unique customs and practices. One of these is the removal of the uvula in babies because of the belief that it may swell up and cause suffocation, even death. The procedure itself is usually done by a traditional, nonbiomedical healer within the community known as an *ankar korach*. Unfortunately, little if any attention is given to sterile technique when performing the procedure, so complications such as tetanus and other bacterial infections, sepsis, and even death can result. The practice is very common in parts of Ethiopia, with one study from 1990 finding that 86 percent of babies in Gondar had had their uvulas removed. The practice is also common among the Bedouin of the southern Sinai Peninsula.[1]

Sarah was in urgent need of IV fluids, antibiotics, and surgical drainage of the abscess that had formed in her palate. I explained this to her father, along with my concerns about how sick Sarah was, and told him that I was not at all certain she'd survive. As the parents returned to the waiting room, I carried Sarah into the treatment room. On my way in, I asked one of the nurses, Tatiana, if she could help me place the IV line, get cultures, and start the fluids and antibiotics.

Tatiana was in her early fifties and had been working in the pediatric emergency room for more than twenty years since moving to Israel from Moscow in the early 1970s. She was excellent at what she did, had a sharp eye for identifying kids whose condition demanded immediate attention, and was very good at making sure that we, the physicians working with her, provided it without becoming distracted by others whose needs were less urgent. She was unflappable and had a great sense of humor.

With the sharp smell of diarrhea still hanging in the air from the last kid who'd been in the treatment room, Tatiana started preparing the IV set, flushes, and adhesive tape while I gingerly lay Sarah down on the treatment bed. Giving her the once-over, Tatiana grimaced and said: "This one looks sick. And dry. Are you going to give her a twenty cc/kg push first?"

Yes, I answered. I quickly explained Sarah's problem to her and what we needed to do. Eyes narrowing slightly, Tatiana took a tongue depressor and flashlight and looked in the child's throat herself. "How awful!" she exclaimed, shaking her head. And then, uncharacteristically, Tatiana fell silent.

Tatiana and I worked quickly, getting the IV fluids and antibiotics in—and the bodily fluids for culture out—in under twenty minutes. Once we had finished the initial procedures and treatments and I had spoken with the surgeon about taking her to the operating room for drainage of the abscess, Tatiana and I made our way over to the break room, she for a smoke, I for a cup of coffee. After taking a long first drag from her cigarette, she exhaled slowly and stared at the glowing ember for what must have been half a minute before looking up at me.

"How could they do that to a three-week old? What exactly was the point?" asked Tatiana. It was a rare display of outrage from her, which said a lot, given the kinds of things we frequently saw in the emergency room. "That baby should be put up for adoption and the parents thrown in jail. What they did to her is an absolute crime!"

I, too, was very disturbed by how sick Sarah was and by how unnecessary it all seemed. Still, I couldn't help but recall an eight-day-old boy

I had cared for just a few weeks earlier. His midmorning arrival to the emergency room had been heralded by the crash of both doors as they burst open and slammed into the walls on either side of the entranceway. He was swaddled in a blue piqué cotton blanket and clutched tightly within the burly arms of his grandmother, her feet seeming not even to touch the ground as she practically flew in. The other three grandparents and the baby's father, all dressed up like they'd just come from a wedding, followed closely behind, each paler than the next. It turned out that something had gone wrong at the baby's *brit mila* (or *bris*, the ritual circumcision that Jewish boys undergo on their eighth day of life in fulfillment of the biblical commandment [Genesis 17:10–14]), and he wouldn't stop bleeding. Thanks to the skillful placement of a suture by one of the urologists on duty that morning, that particular baby did just fine, but I couldn't help contrasting the matter-of-fact "stuff happens" acceptance everyone working that day had displayed toward the baby with the botched *bris* with Tatiana's outrage about what had happened to baby Sarah. Both procedures were, after all, elective surgeries performed on infants in accordance with cultural or religious tradition, both had turned out badly, and neither had been medically necessary, at least not in the conventional sense.

"Why not just stick with normal things, like circumcision?" I asked Tatiana, wondering if she'd pick up on the sarcasm.

She didn't.

"Exactly!" she hissed, shaking her head.

NORMAL AND ABNORMAL

People from different cultural backgrounds often have widely disparate ideas about what constitutes normal and abnormal in all that pertains to health and disease and about how to remedy conditions of disease. This variability has its roots in fundamental differences among traditions, cultural outlook, and worldviews, which in turn are often molded by how individuals and societies are shaped by their environments and socioeconomic circumstances. In this chapter, I'll explore how these differences can detrimentally affect the communication and interaction between physician and patient and lead to either inappropriate or suboptimal care.

Returning to the fundamental role of the physician, namely, the preservation and restoration of health and the alleviation of pain and discomfort, it is very important to understand how we define health and disease. Distinguishing between the two and between trivial and nontrivial instances of disease are, after all, two main reasons why people consult with physicians in the first place. A woman who discovers a lump in her breast has no way of knowing whether it is benign or malignant. To do so she consults with a physician, who draws upon his own experience and that of his colleagues, runs tests, and interprets them accordingly. He then provides her with a diagnosis and offers either a treatment plan or simple reassurance that nothing further needs to be done.

Sometimes, during a routine examination, a physician may diagnose and want to begin treating a patient for a disorder such as glaucoma, for example, which the patient had not only been previously unaware of but which until then had caused him no discomfort or symptoms. Yet treatment is necessary because of the risk of damage to the optic nerve and the potential for irreversible vision loss. Making the diagnosis and initiating treatment require that the physician have both clinical experience and familiarity with objective definitions of health and disease. In the case of glaucoma, this would mean recognizing at what point and beyond the increased intraocular pressure poses a risk to the optic nerve. But just how objective are these "objective" definitions?

The answer to this deceptively simple question turns out to be much more complicated than might first appear. According to the World Health Organization (WHO) "health is a state of complete physical, mental, and social well-being and not merely the absence of disease or infirmity."[2] This isn't very helpful, to put it mildly. As utopian as it is unattainable, the overarching inclusiveness of this definition renders it essentially meaningless. Is it even possible to find anyone on this planet who exists in "a state of complete physical, mental, and social well-being?" The subjectivity implicit in the first half of this statement defies attempts to define objective measures of what does or does not constitute "disease or infirmity," the presence of which would otherwise be taken as evidence of the absence of health.

For most people, however, health actually *is* the absence of disease, whether defined objectively or subjectively. For example, dyspnea, the medical term for shortness of breath, is defined as "a variety of sensations experienced when breathing feels uncomfortable, labored, and unsatisfying."[3] That's it. Most of us breathe more than twenty thousand times each day without even noticing, which is exactly how it ought to be. Becoming aware of your breathing—except, perhaps, in the context of mindfulness training—is a sure sign that something is not right, in the same way as not being aware of your breathing is totally appropriate.

For physicians to provide their patients with good care, it is of paramount importance that there be agreement on what does and does not constitute disease. Should one thousand colony-forming units of bacteria per milliliter of a clean-catch urine sample suffice to diagnose a urinary tract infection, or should one hundred thousand? (The consensus is that it's the latter.)[4] When disease is characterized as something that can be measured or quantified, such as a certain concentration of bacteria in the urine, decreased lung function, or the presence of a tumor, the parameters for when to treat also need to be clearly defined. This is so that interventions can be made in those who are most likely to gain from them while at the same time avoiding the overtreatment of others who will most probably not benefit. Overtreatment can result in pain, disability, and emotional strain and wastes valuable resources that could be better used elsewhere.

While defining disease might appear to be an easy task in that these are, after all, ostensibly well-defined conditions in human beings sharing the same anatomy, physiology, and so on, there is, in fact, significant disagreement between physicians about what does and does not constitute disease, even in the presence of the same symptoms and/or objective findings. Each of us, as a unique biological organism, possesses myriad individual characteristics, some of which invariably fall outside those commonly seen or beyond the range of two standard deviations from the mean. Human variability extends as far as there are humans, and most of it is normal. The arbitrariness with which certain clusters of signs, symptoms, and complaints constitute disease is nowhere more evident than in the marked variability in the very definitions of disease used by the biomedical establishments of different countries.

Addressing a (presumably fictional) newly appointed medical marketing manager of a pharmaceutical company responsible for the European Common Market in an essay in the *British Medical Journal*, M. N. G. Dukes wrote (tongue more than slightly in cheek) about the importance of recognizing the regional variation of medical practice within Western Europe: "You will find that on one side of a frontier cellulitis means muscular rheumatism, and on the other it involves purulent inflammation of the subcutaneous tissue; a hundred kilometers further on it is a euphemism for obesity in puffy young women. Plenty of people are still dying from diseases which other people do not believe in."[5]

Lynn Payer, a former editor of the *New York Times Good Health* magazine, wrote her book *Medicine and Culture* after living and working in Europe as a health journalist. While there, she became keenly aware of how differently the same collections of symptoms were understood and interpreted by physicians in France, England, Germany, and the United States. In all four countries, Western biomedicine was accorded the same elevated status relative to other healing disciplines, and in all four, physicians believed they were adhering to the highest standards of practice. Realizing that the differences in diagnoses stemmed from differences in cultural perceptions of what constituted impaired health, which then translated into fundamental differences in medical practice, Payer wrote:

I began to look at American medicine differently. Many of the practices I had taken for granted now seemed to be not so much the result of scientific progress but rather outgrowths of American cultural biases that in some cases harmed more than helped our health and well-being. In seeing how another country's cultural prejudices affected its medicine, I found it easier to perceive how our own prejudices affect our practice of medicine.[6]

Despite the globalization and the interconnectivity that have allowed for the rapid and widespread dissemination of information in all that relates to the practice of medicine, significant regional variability in how disease is defined and acted upon remains strong. For example, a recent article in the *New York Times* highlighted the differences between how chronic fatigue syndrome (CFS) is defined in the United States, Canada, and Britain and the effects that this has had on both the treatment and prognosis of patients in these countries. The British criteria for CFS, based mostly on the presence of debilitating fatigue lasting for more than six months, are much more inclusive than either the American or the Canadian criteria. When the British criteria were used for a study that found that exercise and cognitive-behavioral therapy were effective in helping people with CFS, the findings were criticized by many North Americans because they were not stringent enough to exclude those patients whose fatigue was caused by depression.[7]

Determining whether or not children with neurodevelopmental delay fall on the autism spectrum is another example of how diagnosis is influenced by societal attitudes about what is normal. As described in a recent article published in *Developmental Psychology*, there are widely disparate rates of autism-spectrum disorder (ASD) diagnosis in different countries. The prevalence rates per ten thousand children range from 1.4 in Oman to 260 in South Korea (2011). In the United States, the Centers for Disease Control and Prevention (CDC) reported in 2012 that the prevalence of ASD was 113.6 for every ten thousand children, one out of every eighty-eight.[8]

Some of the differences in the ASD-diagnosis rates among different societies may be attributed to differences in access to medical and diagnostic services, genetic predisposition, the presence of environmental triggers, and differences in parental age. However, it is also quite likely that the degree of social acceptance of children with developmental delays by their immediate and extended families—and by their school systems—varies significantly among societies. In some, the expressions of psychosocial-developmental delay may be seen more as variation in personality than as the manifestation of a medical disorder, especially when the child has one of the more subtle forms.

One indication that this may be the case is the wide variability of ASD diagnosis made in different regions *within* the United States. According to the 2012 CDC press release, 47.6 out of every ten thousand children in Alabama were diagnosed with an ASD versus 212.7 in Utah, more than a fourfold difference. Likewise, African American and Hispanic children were reported to have had the highest increase in ASD diagnosis since the previous report was issued. It is quite possible that this increase is the result of increasing awareness of ASD within these particular demographics—still much lower than that of the general population,[9] especially within Hispanic households where the primary first language is Spanish—which in turn has led to increased pressure by these parents to have their kids screened. According to the CDC, the prevalence rates of ASD per ten thousand children were 120 for Caucasians, 102 for African Americans, and seventy-nine for Hispanics.[10] Still, if what you as a parent are seeing in your child seems "different" as opposed to "abnormal," and that perception is reinforced by the social circles in which you move and educate your child, you may be less inclined to seek medical attention than if you believe that something is fundamentally wrong with your child.

The same diagnostic variability that exists within the United States regarding neurodevelopmental disorders in children can be found with other conditions as well. One of these is attention deficit and hyperactivity disorder (ADHD). In 2005 the Centers for Disease Control reported that ADHD was diagnosed more than 2.2 times as often in Alabama as it was in Colorado, with prevalence rates of 11.1 percent and 5 percent, respectively. Likewise, the percentage of children being medicated for ADHD varied significantly among the states: 2.1 percent of children in California were on medications for ADHD compared with 6.5 percent in Arkansas, more than a threefold difference.[11]

Because there are such strong subjective components to how ADHD is diagnosed and in how developmentally delayed children are identified as having an ASD and therefore brought to medical or other attention, one might think that there would be less variability in conditions that present with objectively abnormal physical findings. However, here too one can find many examples of diagnostic and therapeutic variability.

A recent review that examined the differences in how esophageal and gastric diseases are determined and defined among different countries found significant disagreement among European, American, and Japanese gastroenterological societies. These differences pertained to how certain malignancies should be classified, which in turn directly influences decisions about further diagnostic workup and treatment. Not only that, it turned out that there was even disagreement about the boundaries of one of the major anatomical landmarks used in their diagnosis, the lower-esophageal sphincter. The authors concluded dryly that "an exchange of views among gastroenterologists in North America, Europe, and Japan would be desirable."[12] So much, then, for the supposition that the science of medicine rests upon solid, incontrovertible, and universal truths.

Even when consensus exists among physicians, it is often short lived. In medical school, our professors made frequent reference to "medicine's pendulum," which swings among different paradigms at regular intervals, whenever one of the students would seem overly dogmatic about how a particular patient should be treated. And indeed, a recent analysis of 363 articles testing established "standards of care" that were published in the *New England Journal of Medicine* between the years 2000 and 2010 found that the results were almost evenly split with regards to their utility. Forty percent found the standard practice to be unbeneficial or even harmful, 38 percent found it to be beneficial, and 22 percent were inconclusive.[13]

Perhaps no better testament to the shaky foundations upon which medical diagnoses are built is the contrast between the working diagnoses made by physicians treating living patients and the final diagnoses made by pathologists after the patient has passed. A large meta-analysis published in 2005 found a 30 to 63 percent disagreement rate between working diagnoses and actual causes of death found on autopsy. Half of all autopsies revealed findings that had not been suspected prior to death. Another study in Britain found that one-quarter of death certificates stated an incorrect cause of death.[14]

Even the very definition of death continues to elude consensus among physicians, as surprising as this might seem.[15] One would think, after all, that determining whether a person is no longer alive should be very straightforward because of death's irreversibility. However, the concept of brain death, upon which much of organ transplantation relies, remains hotly debated, sometimes even among physicians practicing in the same department. It is also worth pointing out that in the ongoing debate about when life begins, with all of the implications that this has on stem-cell research and abortion, the range of opinions held by physicians mirrors that of the general public.

Differences in medical culture directly influence therapeutic decision making, with physicians in one country treating the same clinical problem differently than those in another, even though in both, physicians do so with the same degree of conviction that they are doing what is best for their patients. Take, for example, the issue of caesarean section (CS) versus vaginal deliveries. In 1985 the WHO stated that "there is no justification for any region to have CS rates higher than 10–15 percent." However, a quarter-century later, a study published by the WHO revealed much higher rates of CS than that in many developed countries. In Japan the CS rate was 17.8 percent, in France 18.8 percent, in the United States 30.3 percent, and in Brazil 45.9 percent. By comparison, the infant mortality rates per thousand live births in 2011 for these same countries were 2.21 in Japan, 3.37 in France, 5.98 in the United States, and 20.5 in Brazil. Even when the almost 20 percent home-birth rate in Brazil is taken into account (all of which are vaginal deliveries), both CS and infant mortality rates remain extremely high in that country relative to others.[16] The reason it is important to compare these data side-by-side is because fetal distress is often used as a criterion for proceeding to CS delivery, to prevent harm to the unborn child. Based upon these data, however, one could be forgiven for inferring that increased numbers of CS (including the unnecessary ones) correlate with increased infant mortality.

This variability of practice across societies also holds true as well for vaginal deliveries by women who had previously delivered by CS. According to that same 1985 WHO statement, "there is no evidence that caesarean section is required after a previous caesarean section birth. Vaginal birth after a caesarean (VBAC) should normally be encouraged wherever emergency surgical intervention is available." Yet in 2004, the VBAC rate in the United States was just 9 percent, the lowest of all industrialized countries, less than *one-sixth* that of Holland.[17]

No one would suggest that a physician's decision to take a woman in labor to the operating room for CS is made lightly. It is the result of a complex medical decision-making process based much more upon the subjective interpretation of a large amount of clinical information and circumstance than it is upon cold data. (It is true, however, that there are often additional factors that influence this decision, such as patient preference because of cosmetic reasons and/or a desire to avoid the physical pain of childbirth.) The bottom line, though, is that CS rates in excess of those outlined by the WHO do not provide better outcomes. That being the case, and with the average cost of CS deliveries in the United States almost 70 percent higher than that of vaginal deliveries,[18] as well as the potential for surgical complications, one needs to question the underlying cultural assumptions among physicians that lead them to push for more women to have repeat CS. These differences in the culture of medicine as practiced in different locales extend to institutions as well, with a recent comparison of CS rates in 593 American hospitals revealing rates that ranged from 7.1 to 69.9 percent, an almost tenfold difference![19] In this case, it is not merely the culture of society that influences the practice of medicine but local culture—general and medical—as well.

More evidence of how the local culture of the practice of medicine directly influences treatments proposed by physicians and accepted by patients can be found in a study published in the *New England Journal of Medicine*, which found that American women living in New England were more than 4.5 times more likely to undergo hysterectomy than Norwegian women and almost 2.5 times more likely than English women. This finding led Angela Coulter, Martin Vesey, and Klimt McPherson (McPherson was one of the authors of the *New England Journal* paper) to ask six years later: "Do British women undergo too many or too few hysterectomies?" More recent data published by the OECD in 2012 continue to confirm this discrepancy, with European transvaginal hysterectomy rates per hundred thousand women ranging between twenty-seven in the UK and 243 in Finland, a ninefold difference.[20]

Each of these examples provides insight into the malleability of medical diagnosis—and the practices that derive from it—across societal and cultural lines. Together, they demonstrate how the cultural milieu within which physicians practice exerts a strong influence on how they understand what is presented to them, verbally and nonverbally, by their patients and their caregivers as well as what they, in turn, reflect back and communicate to their patients as far as care and treatment recommendations are concerned.

Recognizing the cultural variability of the supposedly objective basis of Western biomedicine is important for a number of reasons. It can help physicians become more open-minded when dealing with patients who may be accustomed to different treatment approaches for a given condition and who do not understand why what they are now being offered—or simply told to do—is so different from what they are used to. Consider, for example, an American woman who had delivered her first two children via CS in the United States and upon moving to Oslo is told that she will be expected to deliver her third child vaginally. If the recommendation to deliver vaginally is framed in a way that acknowledges the differences in medical practice between Norway and the United States while emphasizing the advantages of vaginal over caesarian delivery, she may well be inclined to agree with and accept the advice of her Norwegian physicians. If, on the other hand, her questions are dismissed with something along the lines of "American doctors don't keep themselves up to date on the latest medical science and are mostly motivated by how much money they can make doing unnecessary procedures," she may well wind up returning to the United States on the first plane back.

In a broader sense, too, recognizing the variability of medical practice can instill in physicians an openness that extends far beyond the narrow scope of diagnosis and treatment by algorithm and results in greater attention being paid to the subjective experience of disease as experienced by the patient, or *illness*, which I'll explore in greater depth in the next chapter. By reminding themselves of just how relative the science of Western biomedicine is, physicians may become more nuanced practitioners of the *art* of medicine, which places the individual patient at the center of attention. This, instead of focusing exclusively on the *science* of medicine, with its standards of practice that are derived from studies of large cohorts of patients with similar constellations of symptoms and findings and that may be absolutely the wrong thing for the particular patient sitting across from them in clinic.

The French philosopher Michel Foucault addressed this dichotomy in his book *The Birth of the Clinic*. Foucault theorized that the categorization and codification of clinical medicine into a scientific corpus of knowledge (*le savoir*) has come at the expense of the undirected "clinical gaze" (*le voir*), with which an individual patient is assessed and examined by an individual physician who is free of outside (empiric) influences that might prejudice the outcome of the clinical interaction.[21] It is important to stress that empiric, population-derived data can be—and are—very useful in determining which treatment has the highest likelihood of successfully treating a specific condition, and such data allow the physician to draw upon the collective experience of his professional community. Yet, if a physician *always* favors the former, rigidly prescribing treatments based solely upon what works for an aggregate of many people with similar symptoms and findings, he risks promoting treatments that are fundamentally unsuited and inappropriate for that particular patient. A fine balance needs to be struck between Foucault's *savoir* and *voir* so that treatment can be tailored to the individual, taking into consideration her personal idiosyncrasies and needs.

RECOGNIZING DIFFERENT FRAMEWORKS OF DISEASE CONCEPTUALIZATION

Just as two physicians from different cultures may understand and interpret the same constellation of objective findings of disease differently, so, too, may the physician and patient not share the same underlying conceptualization of the cause(s) of the patient's disease. This is very important, as there are many instances in which the patient's understanding of his disease differs radically from that of his physician, and that difference may incorporate cultural, religious, and existential components.

The medical anthropologists Merrill Singer and Hans Baer have divided the belief systems within which disease is contextualized into the natural and supernatural. Natural causes of disease include "infection, stress, decrepitude, accident, overt human aggression." To these one could also add misaligned energy flows and bad humors. Supernatural causes of disease include astrology, eloquently described by Daniel Defoe in *A Journal of the Plague Year*: "The wizards . . . always talked to [the people] of such and such influences of the stars, of the conjunctions of such and such planets, which much necessarily bring sickness and distempers, and consequently the plague." Other theories of supernatural disease causation described by Singer and Baer include "fate, ominous sensation, contagion, mystical retribution . . . soul loss, spirit aggression . . . sorcery, [and] witchcraft."[22]

Disease is experienced by the person suffering from it as a series of interlinking events and processes, all of which influence its course, diagnosis, and treatment. The patient becomes aware of her disease and interprets and contextualizes her experience(s) of it within existing frameworks of past experience, personal and societal worldviews, and emotional and psychological states of mind. All serve as filters and lenses through which various components are emphasized, deemphasized, or ignored altogether. The patient then shares her conceptualization of her disease with her physician, who must then process it through his own prisms of conceptualization—personal as well as professional—and in turn reflect them back to her, along with his analysis (the diagnosis) and treatment recommendations.

How patients and their families, physicians, and society at large understand the causes of disease directly influences how they deal with them. They also influence the degree to which the patient will be willing to accept and follow the physician's advice on how best to cure the disease. These perceptions do not arise in a vacuum. Rather, they derive from the larger cultural context of the surrounding society, which may or may not be identical to the physician's. When there is disagreement between the conceptual frameworks employed by physician and patient to explain the disease, its cause(s), and the preferred treatment(s) for it, communication between the two becomes stifled, and misunderstanding and mistrust can easily develop.

For example, a patient who believes that his impotence has been caused by a spell cast by a jealous adversary may respond disdainfully to his physician's suggestion that he lose twenty pounds and pay closer attention to his blood-sugar levels. Similarly, a person with chronic allergies who consults with a practitioner of Eastern medicine after mistakenly thinking that she is a biomedical physician might react scornfully to her suggestion that he undergo acupuncture to correct his blocked energy flows, instead of prescribing nasal steroids or antihistamines.

Anne Fadiman's book *The Spirit Catches You and You Fall Down* describes the collision between the immigrant Hmong parents of Lia Lee, a young girl with refractory epilepsy complicated by poor medical adherence, and the American medical team who tried to care for her. Lia's parents understood Lia's seizures to be caused by soul loss, which occurred during her infancy when her older sister slammed a door inside the family's home, and not by abnormal electrical activity within her brain, as her physicians explained. As a consequence, Lia's parents were reluctant to give her the antiseizure medications prescribed by her physicians, which they not only felt were adversely affecting her behavior but suspected might actually be *causing* her to seize. When Lia's seizures did not completely respond to her medications, her parents stopped giving them to her altogether. This led to longer and more frequent and intense seizures and ultimately culminated in tragedy.[23]

There is no reason that two belief systems, each explaining the circumstances of a particular disease in completely different ways, cannot coexist. And indeed, it can be very counterproductive when physicians insist that their biomedical explanations be granted exclusivity. The curt dismissal of a patient's beliefs by her physician can alienate the patient and cause her to withdraw from the physician and whatever it is he may have to offer her. This is especially true when the biomedical paradigm used to explain and treat the disease process is anything less than completely satisfactory, as was the case with Lia Lee.

Talking with Fadiman, Lia's father said:

> The doctors can fix some sicknesses that involve the body and blood, but for us Hmong, some people get sick because of their soul, so they need spiritual things. With Lia it was good to do a little medicine and a little *neeb* [a shamanic ritual involving animal sacrifice and the exchange of the sacrificial animal's soul for that of the patient whose illness has been caused by soul loss] but not too much medicine because the medicine cuts the neeb's effect. . . . But the doctors wouldn't let us give just a little medicine because they didn't understand about the soul.[24]

Crafting a treatment plan that would have taken both the biomedical and the shamanistic explanatory models into account might have brought Lia's parents around to better adherence with the biomedical treatment her physicians were advocating for, without making them feel devalued and disparaged. And indeed, there is ample evidence that patients who use complementary and/or alternative medicine do not have lower rates of adherence with conventional biomedical treatment. If anything, the opposite is true. The success rates of treating alcoholism among Native Americans, for example, are higher when traditional practices and spirituality are incorporated into the treatment framework.[25]

Michal Shaked and Yoram Bilu, of the Hebrew University of Jerusalem, interviewed the ultra-orthodox Jewish-Israeli parents of thirty autistic children. They found the existence of "a dual system of illness perception in which medical-biological and spiritual-religious frames of references coexist." This duality allowed the parents to receive guidance from religious leaders within their communities as well as from health-care providers who were not members of their communities but whose services they nonetheless required. One mother told the researchers that she "explained the situation to [her son's physicians]: 'he has autistic features, he doesn't talk, please treat him quickly. If I had said that he was possessed by a spirit, would they have understood me? So I termed it as the doctors did.'"[26]

In this case, the patient's mother felt a need to translate how she understood her son's disease into metaphor that was accessible to his physicians because she judged them unable to comprehend her conceptualization of his disease, which was based upon a belief system they did not share with her. And this happens often enough: patients, after all, have just as much experience interacting with other people as physicians do, and they are just as able to intuit when a communication chasm needs to be bridged and when one framework of contextualization needs to be substituted for another. However, even when this strategy is pursued by the patient, it may be limited to outward expression while remaining absent as far as reception and internalization go. The patient may be able to convey his concerns using biomedical metaphors but be unable to understand the physician when he replies in kind. In many ways, this situation is similar to that of an American tourist in Tokyo who cannot speak Japanese and instead relies upon a Japanese phrase book. Although he might be able to ask haltingly for directions to the train station, he is likely to be utterly incapable of understanding the response if it is given in anything other than pantomime.

Shaked and Bilu found that while the ultraorthodox Jewish-Israeli parents they interviewed readily sought the help of medical professionals for their children's care, the position of the physicians in the overall hierarchy of authority was very clear:

> When medical and rabbinical recommendations clash, the mothers will typically adopt the spiritual leaders' advice, despite the priority granted to doctors in the health seeking process. . . . While accepting modern medicine as the main source of knowledge and assistance, they did not receive this knowledge without reservations. . . . One mother conveyed this difficulty as follows: "He recently started saying a few words. In school they work with the PECS [Picture Exchange Communication System technique] . . . I don't know who should I thank for the fact that he now speaks a little. The PECS technique? Or the blessing we got from [the rabbi]? We say that it is all due to our prayers." This somewhat vague conclusion reflects a recurrent theme in the interviews: while professional treatment programs rank higher than spiritual interventions in the ultraorthodox mothers' hierarchy of resort, the mothers tended to attribute greater success to the religiously based interventions.[27]

Shaked and Bilu concluded that when there were conflicts between treatment recommendations made by physicians and those made by the parents' rabbis, the rabbis' recommendations were given much greater weight. "Ultraorthodox parents always follow their rabbis' advice, even on issues that may seem purely medical: The doctors already know of this. They are aware of the fact that . . . [parents] always consult rabbis first. [The doctors] don't like it but that's the way it is."[28]

While maneuvering between parallel belief systems may seem cumbersome, even humiliating to some physicians—particularly those who see themselves at the vanguard of scientific and medical knowledge—it is often essential to achieving the ultimate goal of providing the best possible care to the patient.

Elsewhere in *The Spirit Catches You and You Fall Down*, Anne Fadiman describes how John Aleman, a family physician in Merced, once succeeded in convincing the parents of a sick Hmong infant to agree to a blood draw by contacting a Western-educated Hmong leader: "[The physician] called the head of the family's clan; the head of the clan called the father's father; the father's father called the father; the father talked to the mother; and, having thus received the request through a familiar and acceptable hierarchy, the parents were able to back down without loss of face."[29]

I, too, have had similar experiences. It was not uncommon during my pediatrics residency in Israel for me to have to speak with rabbis about children under my care in order to secure permission to do lumbar punctures in cases of suspected meningitis, or to initiate treatments for certain conditions when their ultraorthodox parents didn't feel comfortable making these decisions on their own. To their credit, I was always impressed by how genuinely and deeply the rabbis with whom I spoke cared about the children of their followers. They were invariably respectful of me and my time and never once made me feel as though their approval of my medical request was somehow arbitrary. (As an aside, it is hard not to compare those conversations with the ones I now often need to conduct with anonymous clerks at health-insurance companies in order to obtain prior authorization for necessary medical testing or treatment for my patients and that often leave me feeling humiliated and frustrated.)

Programs geared to foster a new openness toward other belief systems are already being implemented in many places across the United States. A 2009 article in the *New York Times* described a program at Mercy hospital in Merced, California—the same hospital where Lia

Lee had been a patient years before—which allowed shamans to take an active role in caring for their Hmong patients. Had such a program existed at the time Lia Lee was a patient, it might have altered her parents' decision to discontinue giving her the antiseizure medicines her physicians had prescribed. In that article, Dr. John Paik-Tesch, the director of the Merced Family Medicine Residency Program, described the program as having "built trust both ways."[30]

Still, not everyone reacted favorably to this program. The article in the *New York Times* drew a sharp, almost sarcastic response from Jennifer Hirsch and Emily Vasquez of Columbia University:

> Cultural sensitivity is certainly an improvement over cultural insensitivity. Any real commitment, however, to improving immigrant health would start by considering the critical role of immigrant workers in our economy and the logical corollary that those contributions ought reasonably to be rewarded with the right to purchase health insurance. . . . "Certified shamans" are fine, but the majority of immigrants would be better served by attention to the living and working conditions that put their health at risk and by a less hypocritical conversation about their exclusion from the health care system.[31]

Hirsch and Vasquez seemed to be saying that it's fine to cater to the spiritual needs of immigrants so long as this isn't used as a cover to force them into accepting an objectively inferior system of healing (relative to biomedicine) because of lack of choice and economic realities. Their argument is therefore more about access to affordable health care being a basic human right than about whether or not parallel belief systems should be admitted into those temples of biomedicine, hospitals. However, it is germane to this discussion in that it stresses how important it is not to give up on providing access to state-of-the-art health care to all, including to those whose belief systems are altogether different than the principles of biomedicine.

THE INFLUENCE OF SOCIOECONOMIC DISPARITIES ON PHYSICIAN-PATIENT COMMUNICATION

Even when socioeconomic disparities between physician and patient are not glaringly obvious, they can and often do heavily influence the quality of physician-patient communication during the visit as well as its outcomes. Researchers have found that patients from lower socioeconomic backgrounds tend to participate less in medical decision making, which, as I'll describe in greater detail in chapter 7, results in lower adherence and higher overall health-care costs. These patients are also generally provided with less information and socioemotional support by their physicians. In contrast, patients from higher socioeconomic backgrounds tend to be much more involved in the management of their own care. There are many possible explanations for this, including societal boundaries that limit the scope of communication between people of different social stations and differences in education levels that can impede the ability of physician and patient to find a common language.[32] Whatever the reasons, however, the fact remains that some patients are consistently less engaged by physicians than others, with consequent effects upon their participation in defining the parameters of their care and, ultimately, their adherence with the treatment.

Disparities in socioeconomic status can also have profound effects on how disease is contextualized and understood. In some cases, these can lead to active resistance on the part of patients to public-health disease prevention and treatment efforts. Marilyn Nations of Harvard and Cristina Monte of the Federal University of Ceara Medical School, Brazil, interviewed the indigent residents of two *favelas* (shantytowns) that were hit hard by the 1993 cholera epidemic. Their aim was to understand more fully why there had been such a high degree of resistance by the *favelados* to governmental efforts to control the outbreak, such as water purification and the use of prophylactic antibiotics. Nations and Monte confirmed that in many instances the *favelados'* refusal to cooperate with the campaign was a response to a longstanding sense of marginalization and stigmatization, which was potentiated by the use of certain metaphors in the prevention campaign that seemed to blame them for becoming sick in the first place. By rejecting the government-sponsored prevention efforts, the *favelados* were also rejecting the stigma of being made responsible for the epidemic.

Nations and Monte also discovered a heavy reliance by many of the *favelados* upon supernatural protection. This may have been the consequence of their dismissal of the government-led biomedical disease-prevention campaign, fulfilling their need for some form of protection against the cholera. Conversely, it may have been what empowered and emboldened the *favelados* to reject the government's efforts in the first place, making them secure to do so knowing that they could turn elsewhere for salvation. Nations and Monte recommended that traditional healers and laypeople be involved early on in the prevention and treatment of future epidemics and that the use of fear-driven messaging and stigmatizing metaphor be consciously avoided so as not to alienate the intended beneficiaries.[33] Charles Briggs of the University of California, Berkeley, also described similar experiences to those of the *favelados* in Brazil among the indigenous Warao people of Venezuela during an outbreak of cholera in that country at around the same time.[34] This speaks to the connection between how people contextualize conditions of disease within their socioeconomic status and situation, cultural surroundings, and personal experiences. By seeking out the presence of alternative belief systems in parallel to the biomedical among their patients, and by addressing or even embracing them as appropriate, better physician-patient collaboration can be achieved, resulting in better health outcomes.

Paul Farmer, the physician and anthropologist who is also a cofounder of the humanitarian organization Partners in Health, wrote in his book *Partner to the Poor* that "the failure to contemplate social and economic aspects of epidemics stunts our understanding of them."[35] This is especially true with campaigns to prevent the spread of infectious disease, in which success is predicated upon patients having access to a basic degree of resources that, although taken for granted by either physician or the larger biomedical establishment, might remain beyond the reach of the specific patient. Because differences in socio-economic status play an important role in the communication between physician and patient, a patient who lacks the necessary resources to participate in a public-health disease-prevention campaign may be too embarrassed to speak up and bring this to the physician's attention precisely *because* of the socioeconomic disparities between them. This in turn can result in the failure of those efforts, leaving the physician and larger medical establishment wondering what went wrong. It is not dissimilar to the shame that prevents patients who have difficulty paying for their medications from discussing this with their physicians, as was discussed in chapter 1.

Robert Gilman, of the Johns Hopkins School of Hygiene, and colleagues did a study in the shantytowns of Peru, in which hand-washing practices were observed and knowledge of hygiene tested, in order to determine whether lapses in the former might be explained by deficiencies in the latter and thereby be a contributing factor to the frequent occurrence of diarrheal disease. Gilman found no connection between observed rates of hand washing and whether or not people understood how to maintain good hand hygiene, and he observed a high number of fecal contamination events in the Peruvian shantytowns despite the fact that those involved knew exactly what it was that they were supposed to be doing. These findings contrasted with studies from Bangladesh that had found hygiene-education campaigns to be highly effective in improving hand washing. The difference in behavior between the two populations was explained by the much higher cost of water for washing in Peru, where it was simply too expensive for people to wash their hands even though they knew they should. Lack of knowledge, it turned out, was not the barrier to good health practices. Instead, it was the high cost of adherence. The same failure has been found to occur when people are instructed to boil drinking water with fuel they cannot afford or when the cost of pots and storage containers necessary to treat and store water is beyond their means.[36]

CLOSING THOUGHTS

In this chapter I have described how different belief systems and explanatory models of disease held by physician and patient, as well as socioeconomic differences between the two, can disrupt and complicate the ability of physician and patient to communicate effectively in their quest to achieve the common goal of better health outcomes for the patient. I have explained how important it is that physicians recognize this when trying to engage their patients. In the next chapter I will focus on the subjective components of disease as experienced by the patient, *illness*. I will also explore the triangulation of society, physician, and patient and how both the role of physician and the sick role of the patient, *as defined by society*, can decisively influence the quality of communication between physician and patient.

4

DISEASE, ILLNESS, AND SICKNESS

"For this," he said, "is the great error of our day in the treatment of the human body, that physicians separate the soul from the body."

—Plato

N THE coming pages, I'll explore how the wide range of subjective individual experiences of, and responses to, the same "objective" disease, its associated discomfort, and/or loss of function directly affect how patients interact and communicate with their physicians.

Many scholars distinguish between the objective and subjective aspects of poor health by using *disease* to refer to the former and *illness* to the latter. In his book *Patients and Healers in the Context of Culture*, the psychiatrist and anthropologist Arthur Kleinman defines disease as

> a malfunctioning of biological and/or psychological processes, while the term *illness* refers to the psychosocial meaning and experience of perceived disease. Illness includes secondary personal and social responses to a primary malfunctioning (disease) in the individual's physiological or psychological status (or both).[1]

The substantive differences between objective disease and subjective illness, leaving aside for the moment the elusive nature of disease's "objectivity" as discussed in the previous chapter, were the subject of an essay published by David Jennings in the "Philosophy of Medicine" section of the *Canadian Medical Association Journal*:

One can be seriously diseased without being ill; for example, with silent hypertension or an occult malignant disorder. Conversely, one can be seriously ill without being diseased; for example, with severe depression in response to a loss. Either state can be fatal. It also follows that pain, suffering, and distress are dimensions of illness, not of disease.[2]

Although illness is usually a subjective response to an existing condition of disease, it can also be anticipatory. According to Jeremiah Barondess, a past president of the American College of Physicians:

> Illness . . . is not a biologic, but a human event. It consists of an array of discomforts and psychosocial dislocations resulting from interaction of a person with the environment. The environmental stimulus may be a disease, but frequently it is not . . . it may as readily be a stressful series of life events or a set of reactions to perceived threats which are largely symbolic.[3]

Barondess describes perfectly the circumstances that resulted in Sarah (from the previous chapter) arriving at the emergency room in such a serious condition. Her parents had acted to have her uvula removed because they believed it necessary to prevent a life-threatening condition. They did *not* do so because they were trying to make her conform to certain cultural expectations of their community about appearance, as was the case with foot binding in China in a previous era. Neither did they do so to influence her future sexual behavior, one of the reasons often given to justify female genital mutilation in many societies in Africa and the Middle East.[4] Nor was Sarah's uvula removed in order to fulfill a religious commandment, as is the case with the ritual circumcision of male infants by observant Jews. As seen through mainstream Israeli eyes, Sarah was a completely healthy infant for whom there was no indication for surgery of any kind. Her parents, however, feared that she was at risk of developing a fatal condition that required urgent preemption by a procedure that almost killed her.

From their perspective, the very presence of Sarah's uvula was an illness that needed to be treated.

Even when the objective presentations of disease are the same, the ways in which they are interpreted, understood, and acted upon by different patients can vary dramatically, in accordance with their cultural backgrounds. When on call in the delivery suite in Rehovot, for example, it was very easy for me to guess the ethnicities of the different women in labor based upon how much noise they were making. Ethiopian-Jewish women were invariably the quietest; those of North African descent were usually the loudest. From the hallway it could seem that some women were having a much harder time than others and in greater need of pain relief. Once inside the rooms, however, it was clear that all were more or less uncomfortable to the same degree and that the only real difference was in how loudly they allowed themselves to express their discomfort.

Some, such as Harold Merskey of the University of Western Ontario, have sought to unite the objective aspects of disease with the subjective:

> Disease is a state of malfunction of body or mind that is a matter of concern to the patient, his doctors, and other relevant persons, subject to the qualifications that the malfunction has to be defined from case to case and that the consequences of the disease for the patient's obligations to others (and theirs to him) will be determined by the patient and his doctors with the consent of other relevant persons.[5]

ILLNESS AS BOTH A PERSONAL AND A CULTURAL CONSTRUCT

In his book *Epidemiology and Culture*, James Trostle, of Trinity College, quotes from a speech given by Oliver Wendell Holmes to the Massachusetts Medical Society in 1860, in which Holmes said, "if I wished to show a student the difficulties of getting at the truth from medical experience, I would give him the history of epilepsy to read."[6]

More than a century later, Trostle confirmed this through his own research into how epileptics in Minnesota, Ecuador, and Kenya understood their symptoms and how this understanding informed their sense of illness. Interviewing 127 adults treated for seizures at the Mayo Clinic in Rochester, Minnesota, between the years 1975 and 1980, Trostle found that 79 percent provided distinct biomedical explanations for their symptoms, even though, interestingly enough, their own physicians were only able to establish a definitive cause in 19 percent. Likewise, the majority of patients were able to identify temporal, biomedical, and experiential causes that they felt had triggered their seizures. These included sleep deprivation, stress, and certain emotional states. In contrast, the Ecuadorian epileptics whom Trostle interviewed typically identified "pent-up rage, frustration, suffering and 'nerves' as causes of particular seizures, while they used heredity to explain . . . having seizures in the first place."[7]

The Kenyan epileptics whom Trostle interviewed had still other ways of explaining their seizures. Some identified "malaria, bad blood, and trauma [as well as] cognitive processes such as thinking about problems or imagining things." Others believed that their seizures were contagious, a belief apparently quite common in that community. Trostle noted that one-third of the Kenyan epileptics he interviewed bore scars from burns they had incurred after falling into cooking fires while seizing and not being pulled out quickly enough by onlookers, presumably because the latter feared that the seizures were contagious. Still others felt that their seizures were "supernatural punishment for their misdeeds."[8] Only 13 percent of the Kenyan epileptics acknowledged having epilepsy, compared to the 71 percent who attributed their seizures to malaria. Whether this was because of the overlap that sometimes exists between the two in areas in which malaria is endemic (cerebral malaria can lead to seizures) or because of a desire not to be stigmatized by a disease fraught with negative associations is unclear.

Trostle summarized the findings of his research:

> The influence of culture can be seen in how people care for symptoms before they receive a diagnosis. Groups vary in their willingness to undertake preventative measures; they vary in how they perceive and classify symptoms. Across the world, people employ diverse markers to decide who will be labeled disease-ridden or contagious; they differentially rank which diseases are seen as important or unimportant.[9]

This phenomenon of substituting one diagnosis for another less laden with negative connotations is not uncommon. During my pediatrics residency in Israel, I was frequently approached by the ultraorthodox Jewish parents of children who had been admitted because of seizures, who would ask that I refrain from describing their children's "epilepsy" during rounds. The parents explained that they were concerned that should others learn of their child's diagnosis, it might jeopardize their future chance of a good *shidduch* (an arranged marriage). Similar concerns by Israeli ultraorthodox Jews about the heritability of psychiatric disorders and the potentially negative effects this might have on their offspring's marriage prospects have been described by others.[10]

It may seem obvious that the causes and implications of specific diseases would be experienced and responded to differently by members of well-defined minority groups whose cultural characteristics are easily distinguishable from those of the larger general population. This is also true, however, for members of subgroups within the general population, whose differences in illness behavior are in many instances shaped by cultural differences that may be much less obvious to the physician. These differences can lead to significant variation in how and when people seek care and in how they choose to emphasize or to downplay their symptoms to their physicians. This, in turn, can affect how seriously the complaints are taken by the physician, how extensive a diagnostic workup is pursued, and what treatment recommendations are ultimately made as a result.

ILLNESS BEHAVIOR

David Mechanic, of Rutgers University, has defined *illness behavior* as "the ways in which given symptoms may be differentially perceived, evaluated and acted (or not acted) upon by different kinds of people."[11] Mechanic found that illness behavior can be influenced by the frequency of a disease within a specific population, how familiar members of the population are with its symptoms, the predictability of its outcome, and by how threatening the disease is perceived to be.

A seminal study published in 1966 by C. David Jenkins, a former director of the World Health Organization's Collaborating Center for Psychosocial Factors and Health, on differences in how tuberculosis was perceived by members of different ethnic groups within the United States, demonstrated this graphically. At the time, Jenkins found that African Americans tended to see tuberculosis as "a fast-moving disease which is embarrassing and dirty. . . . Poorly understood scientifically and [which] attacks 'bad people' [rather than] particularly 'good people.'" These attitudes contrasted with how Caucasians and Latinos described tuberculosis, viewing it instead as a "mild, slow-moving, infrequent disease, well understood by medical science . . . [which infects] without regard to the 'goodness' of people." Jenkins noted that the mortality rate from tuberculosis among African Americans at the time of the study was more than double that of Caucasians (down from 3.5 times greater a generation earlier) and thought that this might explain the "reservoir of dread and the emotional and cognitive involvement the Negro associates with [tuberculosis]."[12]

Thirty-two years later, in the mid 1990s, another study was conducted among African American patients with tuberculosis living in some of the poorer neighborhoods of Chicago, to evaluate how their perceptions of illness and its associated stigma affected their behavior. Some patients attributed their disease directly to the decrepit physical condition of their neighborhoods. One interviewee explained that his tuberculosis was caused by: "Garbage, trash, smoking . . . being around a lot of germs."[13] The implications of this cannot be overstated in terms of willingness to adhere with medical treatment: nine months of antibiotic therapy would clearly do nothing to clean up this patient's neighborhood, for example. For this particular patient, the physical environment played a larger role in his conceptual model of his disease than the tuberculosis bacillus itself. This, in turn, would have made it more likely that he would have stopped taking his medications if side effects were to appear, because the meds would "only" be treating the bacillus, which, according to this patient's conceptual model, was a secondary cause, one much less important than his physical surroundings.

Another participant in that particular study confided in the researcher his fears that "if it [tuberculosis] doesn't get treated it could turn into cancer." While tuberculosis is without doubt a serious and potentially life-threatening disease, it is in most cases curable. And even though tuberculosis is still transmissible during the first weeks of treatment, 85 percent of those infected never go on to develop active disease. This stands in stark contrast to the lethality of lung cancer, which has only a 15 percent five-year survival rate.[14] The conflation of the two can result in a fatalistic approach that "no matter what I do," such as taking medications, for example, death is inevitable. It can also provoke deep emotions of shame and guilt as well as fear of killing a loved one through the unintentional transmission of an infection that could potentially transform itself into one of the deadliest forms of cancer. This, in turn, may result in social isolation and withdrawal from the very support networks of family and friends at a time when these are so vitally important in helping the patient to overcome his disease. One patient with tuberculosis described himself simply: "I am a menace. I am a menace."[15]

It therefore becomes clear that the underlying perceptions of disease can have a significant effect on illness behavior. Without open dialogue between physician and patient about how the patient understands her disease, it is very difficult for the physician to identify those concerns that may serve as barriers to effective treatment and to help the patient overcome them. To this end, Arthur Kleinman proposed a model of negotiation between health-care practitioners and patients as a basis for establishing a relationship that addresses and ultimately better serves the needs of the patient. To do so, according to Kleinman, some or all of the following steps need to occur:

1. Explanation of the illness by the patient to the physician
2. Explanation in lay terms, by the physician to the patient, of the biomedical aspects of the disease and its proposed treatment(s)
3. Convergence and alignment of the physician's proposed treatment plan with the expectations and needs of the patient to produce a plan that satisfies both patient and physician; this may require additional negotiation. Note that this convergence addresses both disease *and* illness
4. When this alignment is not possible, the physician should attempt to reach a compromise with the patient about the treatment plan that neither unduly endangers the patient nor undermines the physician's own ethical standards
5. If satisfactory compromise remains impossible, a different physician should be found, either by the patient or the first physician; as Kleinman writes: "It is essential to recognize that the physician's role is to provide expert advice and rationale for treatment recommendations but the patient is the final arbiter of whatever choice is made. . . . The ultimate choice is [the patient's and the patient's family]"
6. The treatment plan negotiated should frequently be reevaluated, renegotiated, and updated as needed[16]

While doing medical volunteer work in Haiti in November 2010, my team cared for an infant born several weeks prematurely who was otherwise well and whom we felt could be discharged home, except for one thing: his mother adamantly refused to nurse him. His chances of surviving on powder-based formula would have been slim because his family lived in one of the many tent cities that had sprung up in Port-au-Prince in the aftermath of the January 2010 earthquake. Cholera had reappeared on the island only three weeks earlier, after a decades-long absence, and was sickening thousands. Access to clean drinking water, a necessary ingredient for preparing infant formula, was unpredictable and unreliable.

Initially, we could not understand this mother's stubborn refusal to nurse, which seemed a frivolous and reckless endangerment of her son's life. However, Denise, the nurse on our team who was caring for the baby, soon learned from his mother that a previous child of hers had died in infancy. At that time, the mother had been told by a *houngan* (a traditional Voodoo priest) that her milk was bad and that were she ever to nurse again, those babies too would surely die.

The belief in *lèt gat* (spoiled milk), which can be harmful to a nursing infant and is itself caused by *move san* (bad blood), a condition arising from physical abuse sustained by a woman at the hands of a partner or spouse, is widespread in Haiti.[7] And indeed, it turned out that these were exactly this young mother's circumstances. She told Denise that she was being regularly beaten by the father of her son.

It took a lot of coaxing to get this mother to nurse her child, and ultimately, what finally made the difference was a conversation between Denise and the infant's maternal grandmother. After the grandmother was satisfied that her daughter's milk was not tainted, she gave her blessing for the mother to express a small quantity of milk into a bottle for her baby. Once the mother saw that no harm befell him she began to nurse him fully, and within a few days we were able to send him home safely, thriving and gaining weight.

In an essay on this topic in his book *Partner to the Poor*, Paul Farmer described an interaction between physician and patient in which "the doctor refused to admit *move san* into the range of his competence, and the patient tacitly agreed to act as if the disorder had never occurred. Doctor and patient were not, therefore, speaking the same language." Unless physician and patient "speak the same language," it is extremely difficult to change illness behavior. As Arthur Kleinman wrote in *The Illness Narratives*:

The illness experience includes categorizing and explaining, in common-sense ways accessible to all lay persons in the social group, the forms of distress caused by those pathophysiological processes. And when we speak of illness, we must include the patient's judgments about how best to cope with the distress and with the practical problems in daily living it creates.[18]

This is true for illness behavior *already being expressed*, such as the refusal of the Haitian mother just described, to nurse because of an alternative belief system dictating that specific behavior (and not, as might have been the case in the West, because of considerations of personal convenience). It is also true of illness behavior that the patient *anticipates he may need to adopt* as a price to be paid for treating the disease and that he does not want to pay, unbeknownst to the physician. For example, a study done by a South African group at the School of Public Health, University of Witwatersrand, looked at how culture-specific beliefs about tuberculosis in that country affected illness behavior. The researchers found that certain beliefs correlated with delays in presentation to medical care and decreased adherence with treatment. These included the belief that tuberculosis was caused by inappropriate behavior instead of by bacteria, thereby rendering it more effectively treated by traditional (nonbiomedical) healers, and the belief that the biomedical treatment would only succeed if patients abstained from sexual relations during the months of antibiotic treatment.[19]

HOW ILLNESS BEHAVIOR AFFECTS
DISEASE PREVENTION

The cultural specificity of illness behavior extends to those factors that enable disease to spread in the first place. The centrality of the cultural determinants of illness behavior to disease prevention, and what happens when these are disregarded or ignored outright by the physician or by the larger biomedical establishment, are well demonstrated by the many failed disease-eradication campaigns of the last decades. Most of these campaigns were designed and implemented by well-intentioned

Westerners without the involvement of local physicians and community leaders, a critical oversight.

For example, many malaria eradication campaigns in Africa and elsewhere have foundered because of differences in disease conceptualization that were not taken into consideration by those who designed and ran them. In her book *The Fever*, Sonia Shah noted that the Chewa people living alongside Lake Malombe in Malawi, Africa, ascribed malaria not just to mosquitoes but to "spirits and jealousy and hexes and bad weather and hard work and dirty water and rotten food, among other things." Small wonder, then, that they quickly gave up sleeping under the insecticide-impregnated nets that had been distributed to them, using them instead to catch fish. Why go to all the trouble of spreading the nets out at night and putting them away the next day, when these were powerless against what they perceived to be the *real* causes of malaria?[20]

Because physicians who emerge from within the communities they serve are more attuned to the cultural attitudes and preconceptions that shape illness behavior, engaging local medical personnel and establishments in the planning and execution of disease eradication campaigns, especially international ones, is vital. However, even that is not always sufficient, and it is often necessary to bring in others in whom the patients have more trust.

In 2004, the *Baltimore Sun* published an investigative report about the collapse of the polio-eradication campaign in Nigeria the previous year, which had resulted in the resurgence of polio in that country as well as its reemergence in neighboring countries it had previously been eliminated from. One of those interviewed was Ibrahim Datti Ahmed, a physician by training and the president of Nigeria's Supreme Council for Sharia Law. Ahmed had initially been active in the anti-polio campaign, even immunizing his own children against the virus. Subsequently, however,

Ahmed concluded that the United States was contaminating the vaccine with anti-fertility hormones to depopulate the developing world, afraid that rapid population growth in countries like Nigeria, with 126 million people, will overwhelm the United States, where birth rates are lower. "They are the worst criminals on Earth to sterilize children for life. Even Hitler was not as evil as that," said Ahmed.[21]

Another Nigerian interviewed observed that "there are more killer diseases that need attention in Africa than polio. Like malaria. It's the No. 1 killer."

The sentiment among members of the target population that the goals of the eradication campaign served the interests of others more than their own is similar to what the anthropologist Svea Closser witnessed and described in her book *Chasing Polio in Pakistan*. Closser identified an enthusiasm gap between the (mostly foreign) physicians overseeing the campaign and the Pakistanis who were the ostensible beneficiaries of it:

> The problem is that polio is not a ranking public health problem in Pakistan. In a country where one in ten children dies before age five, polio now paralyzes fewer than a hundred children each year. Also, polio's status in Pakistan as an endemic, not an epidemic disease means that it does not evoke the fear that it did in the midcentury United States. . . . Polio eradication, which relies on mass vaccination of the entire population, cannot rely on the fear of parents around a single polio case to galvanize nationwide vaccination.[22]

The inability of individual physicians and medical establishments, local and foreign, to distinguish between endemic and epidemic polio derailed their attempts to enlist the collaboration of the local population, which in turn led to the failure of the anti-polio campaign in Pakistan. Without this collaboration, the eradication program was doomed from the start. Its goals became unattainable when the physician organizers and the prospective beneficiaries of the program used the same word, *polio*, to describe two very different diseases, one endemic and the other epidemic, each of which drove radically different illness-behavior responses.

It is useful to contrast what seems like indifference toward *endemic* polio in Africa and Asia with the terror caused by *epidemic* polio in the United States prior to mass vaccination. The disease would sweep into cities without warning in the summertime, leaving hundreds dead and crippled in its wake. Describing one such outbreak in Hickory, North Carolina, in 1944, the historian David Oshinsky wrote in his Pulitzer Prize–winning book, *Polio: An American Story*, "Panic swept the region. Public events were canceled. Swimming pools, movie theaters, and libraries were closed. People drove through the sweltering summer heat of Hickory with their car windows rolled up. Trains sped by. Health officials in neighboring states warned North Carolina residents to stay away."[23]

THE IMPORTANCE OF METAPHOR IN COMMUNICATION BETWEEN PATIENTS AND PHYSICIANS

One of the most common means of translating our own personal experiences and knowledge into concepts that can then be shared with and made accessible to others is through the use of metaphor. This is true, of course, not just for matters pertaining to illness and disease but for virtually every aspect of our daily lives. The choice of a particular metaphor to describe a specific situation or circumstance depends in large part upon the underlying belief systems, culture, and language of the narrator. This is why it is often so difficult for a listener from a different background to understand what is being said by a speaker unless he is familiar with the metaphor being used or unless it is transposed into a different one that conveys with rough approximation the intended meaning. According to the cognitive linguist George Lakoff and the philosopher Mark Johnson, authors of the book *Metaphors We Live By*, "truth is always relative to a conceptual system . . . mostly metaphorical in nature, and . . . therefore, there is no fully objective, unconditional, or absolute truth."[24] Unless we recognize and are able to grasp the meaning of the descriptors in one another's narratives, our ability to effectively communicate is diminished. True with all forms of interpersonal communication, this is especially important in the dialogue between patient and physician, given the stakes involved.

Often, the metaphors people employ to describe conditions of health and illness are easily understood—again, with the caveats of cultural and linguistic relativity. Consider the opening paragraph of *Mortality*, in which Christopher Hitchens describes the moment he first realized that something was seriously wrong with him, that "something" being terminal esophageal cancer:

> Nothing prepared me for the early morning in June when I came to consciousness feeling as if I were actually shackled to my own corpse. The whole cave of my chest and thorax seemed to have been hollowed out and then refilled with slow-drying cement. I could faintly hear myself breathe but could not manage to inflate my lungs.[25]

However, metaphor that is used to explain disease processes within one healing framework can often be unintelligible in another. Example of this include energy flows along meridians, the interaction of humors, the balance of hot and cold, the memory of water, and the consequences of hexes. All may be as incomprehensible to the physician practicing biomedicine as concepts of innate immunity and missense mutations may be to practitioners and adherents of other healing practices. The physician must remember that not every patient comes to him after having been schooled in biomedicine or, for that matter, embraces it at the exclusion of other healing practices and frameworks she is familiar with. Because of this, the metaphor used by the patient to describe what he is experiencing to his physician, as well as how the patient understands the metaphor used by the physician, may be totally different than what he, the physician, might expect. This is especially true as far as somatization goes. Examples of different metaphors used to describe somatic symptoms of anxiety or depression include *dhat*, or loss of vitality ascribed to semen loss, in India; "brain fag" in Nigeria; and "heart distress" in the Middle East.[26]

Metaphor is often used to convey hope, despair, and other emotional states that are part of the subjective illness. The Reverend Mary Robinson, the director of pastoral care at Boston Children's Hospital, once described to me visiting a boy who was undergoing chemotherapy for leukemia. Entering the room, she saw he was wearing a large Red Sox baseball hat that completely covered his hairless head.

"So tell me about your hat," she asked him. He looked at her and said: "I'm a lot like the Red Sox. I never give up, and I'm going to win the Series."

The issue of his hair loss never came up in their conversation: it was beside the point. The hat itself was a touchstone for something much deeper and spiritual.[27]

SICKNESS

Metaphor plays an important role in *sickness*, one more aspect of how the patient experiences disease. Sickness relates to how society defines the unhealthy person and (re)assigns her a role within it, even when she (the patient) does not recognize herself as being unhealthy.[28] Sickness integrates the patient's perception of her own illness with how she is viewed by society and helps both patient and society calibrate their expectations of the new role the patient must assume because of her disease.

Societal attitudes toward disease weigh heavily upon how patients interpret their symptoms and construct the narratives of their illnesses. They also directly influence the way patients are treated by their physicians and by larger society. As I've already discussed, the ways in which disease is conceptualized and either avoided or treated by both patient and physician are strongly influenced by society. This, in turn, can bear heavily upon the communication between the two. A person defined as "sick" is cast into a role that determines how she is regarded by others, including physicians, as well as what responses on her part to her disease may be considered acceptable. Her sick role will also determine which treatment options will be made available to her for remedying her condition, and it may also strongly affect her socioeconomic status going forward.

While this is certainly true for physical forms of disease, it is even more pronounced with mental disorders, especially when the person being given the diagnosis does not accept that he is sick, much less ill or diseased. As the iconoclastic psychiatrist Thomas Szasz wryly put it: "The patient with bodily illness, experiencing suffering, is driven to see a physician by pain [while] the patient with mental illness, making others suffer, is driven to see a psychiatrist by the police. The difference between . . . [them] is like the difference between the ways the word *driven* is used in these two sentences."[29]

Ever since antiquity, certain diseases have been understood to be the well-deserved wages of sin, divine punishment for transgressions. When Miriam, the sister of Moses, mocked him for taking a dark-skinned wife, she was stricken with leprosy and forced to dwell outside of the camp for seven days until it had passed (Numbers 12:1–16). The "uncleanliness" associated with the leprosy was seen by the Israelites as being as much a spiritual as a physical affliction, and, indeed, it was the spiritual transgression that was viewed as the cause of the physical disease meted out to her as punishment. Elsewhere in Numbers (25:1–13), the Bible describes an outbreak of plague that was sent by God to punish the Israelites because of their promiscuity and worship of the Midianite god Ba'al Pe'or during their wanderings in the Sinai desert. In the Book of Psalms (91:6), plague is described as a demon "walking in darkness," stealthily stalking its victims.

More than two millennia later, Daniel Defoe described the plague that ravaged London in 1665 as having "[come] at length to spread its utmost rage and violence in these parts," "like a fire," and as "distemper, eminently armed from Heaven . . . executing the errand it was sent about." This errand, according to Defoe, was punishment. "This dismal time to be a particular season of Divine vengeance. . . . This was a day of visitation, a day of God's anger."[30]

In the United States, attitudes toward patients with AIDS at the onset of the epidemic in the early 1980s were often very hostile. At the time, most were either men who had sex with other men or intravenous drug users, and they commonly were blamed for having become sick as the direct result of what was seen by many as aberrant and immoral behavior. Instead of receiving sympathy, they often were treated with callousness and downright hostility and viewed as somehow deserving of their fate, cast many times in biblical terms. These conceptual frameworks, with their built-in prejudices against people with AIDS in the early years of the epidemic, guided the behavior of some physicians and resulted in implicit—and at times explicit—animosity toward their patients with AIDS.

Ronald Godwin, at the time the executive vice president of the Moral Majority, explained in 1983 to the *New York Times* why he opposed government funding of AIDS research. "What I see is a commitment to spend our tax dollars on research to allow these diseased homosexuals to go back to their perverted practices without any standards of accountability." In the same article, an anonymous doctor from New Orleans was quoted as asking a professor at Tulane University: "Jim, you think God's trying to punish them [homosexuals]? 'Cause if he is, it ain't enough."[31] It doesn't take a lot to imagine how badly the interaction between this physician and a homosexual AIDS patient unlucky enough to have fallen under his care would have gone. And it is also hard to imagine a situation in which the imbalance of power between a dying man desperate for help and a physician believing that the person before him deserves to suffer as punishment for his sins could be any starker.

This particular physician's attitude toward AIDS patients was similar to that of a large segment of American society at the time, as demonstrated in a study that assessed the reactions of psychology students to different patient scenarios. The researchers found that the students' emotional responses (pity, anger, and willingness to help) differed markedly depending upon how a hypothetical AIDS patient had become infected. When infection was described as the result of sexual activity—at the time, synonymous with homosexual relations— the responses were much more negative than when it was described as having occurred because of a transfusion of tainted blood, indicating that the patient been infected through no "fault" of his own.[32]

Over the years, concurrent to the development of effective anti-retroviral treatment, AIDS has evolved, in the United States and other affluent countries, into a disease to be lived with and not necessarily to die from. The transformation in how AIDS is perceived, however, stops conspicuously at the borders of the developed world. It does not, for the most part, extend to developing nations, where millions of patients, especially in Africa, are sick and dying from AIDS because of lack of access to the very medications that have changed the face of AIDS in wealthier countries. There, the metaphors used to describe HIV and AIDS continue to include death, punishment, crime, horror, and a source of shame,[33] resulting in its victims being marginalized and shunned rather than embraced and supported. In *Our Kind of People*, Uzodinma Iweala, a physician who divides his time between the United States and Nigeria, writes that "in Hausa-speaking northern Nigeria, the word for HIV/AIDS is *kanjamau*. This translates roughly as skeleton." An HIV-positive woman in Lagos tells Iweala about her feelings in the aftermath of a sermon at her church: "You go home judging yourself to death: 'Oh, I'm a bad person. I don't even deserve to live in this world. Oh! Nothing good can come of me.'"[34]

Another disease in which societal attitudes and influence are strongly felt is cancer. In 1989, Susan Sontag described her experiences as a cancer patient in her book *Illness as Metaphor and AIDS and Its Metaphors* and wrote about how the negative metaphor affixed to her disease directly affected her and added to the sick role that society had cast upon her: "When I became a cancer patient, what particularly enraged me—and distracted me from my own terror and despair at my doctors' gloomy prognosis—was seeing how much the very reputation of this illness added to the suffering of those who have it. Many fellow patients . . . evinced disgust at their disease and a kind of a shame."[35]

In recent years, at least in the United States, there has been a big shift in how cancer is viewed. Cancer is increasingly portrayed as a foreign invader that "strikes without warning" against which "war" is waged with the goal of either "defeating" or "conquering" it altogether. Individuals stricken with cancer are seen to either "battle and survive" or "lose the fight" and succumb with "bravery."[36] These metaphors convey the respect now given to cancer patients, perceived as noble victims of a malignant outside force against which they mount a valiant struggle. Rarely now is blame leveled at cancer patients for their disease, except, perhaps in cases of primary lung cancer, 90 percent of which can be attributed to smoking.[37]

Not that the reduction in stigma has made the diagnosis of cancer a less fearsome one, even when the prognosis is very good, and it continues to evoke a powerful response as far as illness behavior is concerned. Being told they have cancer can drive some to pursue aggressive, costly, and often unnecessary treatments even when the benefits are questionable at best and associated with increased morbidity and mortality at worst. This often includes surgery to remove organs in which certain forms of precancerous tissue abnormalities have been detected, which may or may not ever evolve into actual disease. Another example is contralateral prophylactic mastectomy in which both breasts, not just the one with the cancer, are removed, even when not medically indicated because of the lack of any proven health benefit.[38] Recognizing the psychological impact that being diagnosed with "cancer" has on illness behavior, an expert panel at the National Cancer Institute recently recommended that certain forms of premalignant disease such as ductal carcinoma *in situ* of the breast and high-grade prostatic intraepithelial neoplasia be renamed so as not contain the words "cancer," "neoplasia," or "carcinoma." The stated goal of this proposal was to try to reduce the anxiety driving unnecessary overtreatment.[39]

All this demonstrates just how important society's definition of sickness is to the person who has been designated as sick, and it speaks to the influence that it has on the physician charged with providing care to the sick patient. The malleability of sickness is much greater even than that of disease, as was discussed in the previous chapter. If we compare two American AIDS patients, one diagnosed in 1985, the other diagnosed in 2005, although they would share the same disease, the manifestations of their sickness, illness, and illness behavior would dramatically different.

Over time, social mores may evolve so dramatically as to render obsolete definitions of sickness that until just a short time ago had seemed unshakeable. However, even after this happens the physician remains bound to her patient and to the ramifications of how she has treated him. It is to the patient, first and foremost, as well as to her own conscience and sometimes even to the new norms that society has adopted, that the physician will be required to answer if and when moral and ethical questions arise. So, as great as the temptation may be at the time to embrace unquestioningly the sick roles defined by society for those who meet their definitions and criteria, the physician is well advised to remain loyal to the patient, his needs, and the voice of her own conscience. In the coming pages I'll present examples of defined sickness that have either disappeared or changed radically, with profound implications for those designated as "'sick" as well as, one hopes, for the physicians involved in their care.

THE MUTABILITY OF SICKNESS

Hysteria was a common diagnosis, peaking in the latter half of the nineteenth century. It was often given to women who presented with a vague assortment of complaints such as lassitude, emotional instability, and abdominal discomfort. The topic of lively debate among such medical luminaries of the time as Jean-Martin Charcot, Sigmund Freud, and Josef Breuer, hysteria was thought to be the consequence of abnormalities of the female reproductive organs (the word *hysteria* comes from *hystera*, Greek for uterus). Hysteria was remedied with a variety of treatments, which in the extreme entailed surgical removal of these same organs. A less radical and more common treatment of hysteria was "pelvic massage,'" performed by the mostly male physicians on their female patients until the latter achieved orgasm. The physicians of the time found providing this treatment distasteful, which ultimately led to the invention of the enduringly popular electro-mechanical vibrator.[40]

Yet despite hysteria being such a commonly diagnosed condition, within the space of a few years it had completely disappeared from the diagnostic lexicon of most physicians. "How," asked the medical historian Mark Micale rhetorically, "have we gotten from the famous belle époque of hysteria in the closing decades of the nineteenth century to the virtual disappearance of the disorder two decades later?" He quoted Charcot's biographer, George Guillain: "In reality, the patients have not changed since Charcot; it is the words to describe them that have changed." Micale then pointed out that the diagnosis of hysteria was supplanted by others that addressed individually, rather than collectively, the different components that together served as its basis, what he called "atomization of the diagnosis."[41]

Although one might argue that in the end it matters little whether a specific person is labeled as suffering from condition A or B, that is, hysteria or chronic anxiety, it is impossible to separate the diagnostic paradigms which generate these labels (A or B) from the therapeutic recommendations that inevitably follow. Many women who were diagnosed with hysteria suffered greatly and unnecessarily, some even dying of complications, when their reproductive organs were surgically removed in an attempt to stabilize their mood.[42] Had these same women presented to their physicians twenty years later with identical symptoms, they would likely have been given another diagnosis and been treated altogether differently, and most certainly nonsurgically.

The transformation over a few short decades of the American biomedical establishment's definition of homosexuality, from a form of mental sickness to a normal biological variant, is an excellent example of the adaptation of biomedicine to larger normative changes within society. It is hard to believe that as recently as 1970 the *Journal of the American Medical Association* published an article by the psychiatrist Charles Socarides in which he referred to homosexuality as "a dread dysfunction, malignant in character, which has risen to epidemiologic proportions." Socarides wrote that homosexuality's "frequency of incidence surpasses that of the recognized major illnesses in the nation" and maintained that "the claim that homosexuality is simply a variant of normal sexual behavior and exists alongside heterosexuality as an equivalent expression of adult sexual maturation is utterly false." Finally, Socarides concluded that "above all, the homosexual must be recognized as an individual who presents a medical problem."[43]

After failing in his attempts to block the American Psychiatric Association (APA) from removing homosexuality as a disorder from the Diagnostic and Statistical Manual of Mental Disorders (DSM) in 1973, Socarides founded the National Association for the Research and Therapy of Homosexuality (NARTH). This is an organization that has and continues to promote the so-called "Treatment of Unwanted Same-Sex Attractions and Behavior."[44] Articles on the NARTH website include one purporting to show that counseling given to homosexual men who had expressed interest in changing their sexual orientation succeeded in "greatly reduc[ing] or [making] non-existent" their "same-sex struggles" in 73 percent of cases.[45]

Robert Spitzer was a psychiatrist instrumental in the APA's 1973 decision to demedicalize homosexuality. This, however, did not prevent him from conducting later research into the role of so-called reparative therapy for homosexuality. One of his studies, in which two hundred homosexual men and women who had undergone such "reparative therapy" for their homosexuality were supposedly found to have changed "from a predominantly or exclusively homosexual orientation before therapy to a predominantly or exclusively heterosexual orientation," was published in 2001.[46] This methodologically problematic study and its findings were roundly attacked and dismissed but nonetheless provided the validation others sought for their efforts to treat homosexuality as a sickness in need of a cure.

Spitzer ultimately wound up publicly apologizing to the gay community in May 2012.[47] That also happened to be the month that Mirta Roses Periago, the director of the Pan-American Health Organization, stated unequivocally:

> These supposed conversion therapies constitute a violation of the ethical principles of health care, and violate human rights that are protected by international and regional agreements. Since homosexuality is not a disorder or a disease, it does not require a cure. There is no medical indication for changing sexual orientation. . . . Practices known as "reparative therapy" or "conversion therapy" represent a serious threat to the health and well-being—even the lives—of affected people.[48]

Completing the transformation of homosexuality from sickness to normal variant, on September 29, 2012, Governor Jerry Brown of California signed into law the first bill of its kind in the United States outlawing conversion therapy of gay children and adolescents. California State Senator Ted Lieu, the author of the bill, was quoted as saying: "These attempts [at reparative therapy] are quackery and this kind of psychological abuse of children must stop."[49]

Precisely because so much of what is considered normal and abnormal by individuals and society is constantly being redefined, and because these very same processes are at work within the subculture of biomedicine, which is by nature more conservative than society at large, definitions of sickness need to be approached with caution and humility by physicians. For example, attempted suicide rates in lesbian, gay, bisexual, and transgender (LGBT) teens are more than five times greater than those of the general teen population and 20 percent higher still among those who live in unsupportive social environments.[50] Many LGBT youth suffer bullying at school, and some are disowned by their families. Physicians can either serve as strong pillars of support for adolescents grappling with their sexual identity or, alternatively, mire them more firmly in despair by keeping in lockstep with entrenched social bias and prejudice. Discussing safe-sex practices in a nonjudgmental way with a seventeen-year-old young man who presents with anal gonorrhea will serve him much better than preaching abstinence or prescribing discredited sexual-orientation reparative therapy.

WHEN PHYSICIANS' SENSE OF OBLIGATION TO SOCIETY SUPERSEDES THEIR LOYALTY TOWARD THEIR PATIENTS

There is a difference between physicians who wear their social prejudices on their sleeves, such as the one described earlier who was so hostile toward AIDS patients, and those who conform to a political ideology that manipulates medicine to harm individuals in the service of its own goals. It was common practice in the former Soviet Union to incarcerate political dissidents in psychiatric institutions, in the absence of any evidence of mental sickness other than political dissent, which served as sufficient "proof" of mental sickness in the eyes of the authorities and the psychiatrists who collaborated with them. Inmates of these psychiatric prisons were "treated" with powerful antipsychotic drugs, insulin comas, and shackled in physical restraints because of "symptoms" that consisted mainly of "'delusions of reform' and 'anti-Soviet thoughts.'"[51]

Richard Bonnie, a professor of law and the director of the Institute of Law, Psychiatry, and Public Policy at the University of Virginia, points out that it is impossible to ascribe this pervasive abuse merely to the corruption of individuals who cast aside their obligations to their patients for the sake of personal, political, or financial benefit. Rather, there was buy-in to this on the part of many Soviet psychiatrists who conflated political ideology with morality, a very dangerous mix. He writes:

The mental health of dissidents could be contested, even if diagnoses were grounded in a single internationally recognized system of classification, but the problem is all the more complicated when psychiatrists in different societies are trained to understand normality and psychopathology in different ways. Taking into account culturally linked ambiguities in psychiatric diagnosis, it seems likely that at least some cases of alleged abuse represent good-faith efforts by psychiatrics to apply prevailing psychiatric knowledge in politically repressive societies.[52]

This echoes what Walter Reich, a psychiatrist and a fellow at the Woodrow Wilson Institute, asserted in an article published in the *New York Times* following a meeting he participated in with Andrei Snezhnevsky, the director of the Institute of Psychiatry of the Soviet Academy of Medical Sciences in 1982. At that time, motions to expel the Soviet All-Union Society of Psychiatrists and Neuropathologists were being brought before the World Psychiatric Association because of the Soviet organization's complicity in the abuses described above.[53] These were not simply a few bad apples. Many, if not most, of the Soviet psychiatrists diagnosing dissidents with mental sickness did, in fact, believe that they were acting in full accordance with accepted professional standards. And again, it is worth pointing out that in the absence of objective criteria of disease, or subjective symptoms disruptive to the patient (illness), these dissidents were being diagnosed with and being treated for a sickness whose only manifestation was political dissent.

It is not surprising, therefore, to learn that the Hippocratic Oath was done away with in the Soviet Union following the 1917 Revolution. As Thomas Szasz wrote, the real conflict between the underlying philosophies of Soviet and Western biomedicine was over the question of to whom physicians owed their supreme allegiance: society or the individual patient.[54] Soviet biomedicine saw the physician as having a greater obligation toward society, whereas Western biomedicine mostly viewed the physician as being ultimately responsible toward the individual patient.

There are, of course, those who continue to challenge the diagnoses of mental sickness made by psychiatrists in democratic societies in individuals who refuse to accept that there is anything the matter with them and who view this as the exercise of political, moral, and social, rather than medical, judgment. In their opinion, the diagnosis of mental sickness and its consequences, which can include forced incarceration and medication, are no more than social control and engineering. Carrying this argument to the extreme, Thomas Szasz held that "there is no medical, moral, or legal justification for involuntary psychiatric interventions. They are crimes against humanity."[55] However, most would agree that there is a significant difference between incarcerating and forcibly medicating individuals who pose an immediate danger to themselves or to others and doing so simply because they are critical of their government's policies.

It is sobering to consider that Reich's article in the *New York Times* even needed to be written almost forty years after the Nazi Doctors' Trial in Nuremberg (1946–1947). That is where twenty-three prominent German physicians were tried for crimes against humanity because of their active roles in the mass torture and murder of millions of Jews and others considered racially and genetically inferior by the Nazi regime. Although the trial focused mostly on crimes committed against Jews and other non-Germans, many Germans suffered as well from the wholehearted embrace by the German biomedical establishment of the murderous Nazi ideology. This enthusiasm was not confined merely to its leaders or to a small number of sadists, ideological fanatics, and political opportunists. It extended to the rank and file as well, and, indeed, 45 percent of German physicians became members of the Nazi party. Their active and passive cooperation with the Nazi regime was instrumental to the success of the campaign of mass sterilization of between three and four hundred thousand Germans deemed "genetically defective." With the outbreak of World War II, the sterilization campaign was supplanted by one of euthanasia, resulting in the murder of more than seventy thousand people in under two years. Included among the victims were more than five thousand children with congenital abnormalities and tens of thousands of adults with psychiatric disorders. According to testimony given by Hans

Hefelmann, the man in charge of the children's euthanasia program, at a trial held in Limburg in 1946: "No doctor was ever ordered to participate in the euthanasia program; they came of their own volition."[56]

German biomedicine during the Nazi period accepted definitions of sickness and sought to eradicate it by means that directly conflicted with the most fundamental of human rights: to live, to enjoy as pain free an existence as possible, and to reproduce. Overriding these basic human rights in the name of society's prerogative to eradicate what it arbitrarily defines as sickness alters the role of physician from one of patient advocate to that of society's agent, in the pursuit of an agenda that can directly conflict with the patient's. Even when the conflict is not as extreme, the physician-patient relationship transforms from a trusting and collaborative one into a potentially adversarial one. Even if that potential is never fulfilled, once apparent, its presence undermines any possibility that the patient can trust his physician, and it forecloses meaningful communication between the two.

The lingering effects of the infamous Tuskegee Syphilis Study conducted by the U.S. Public Health Service continued to be felt for years beyond its conclusion. In this study, almost four hundred African American men infected with syphilis were observed over a forty-year period (1932–1972) without being given treatment even though effective antibiotic therapy had become widely available following the Second World War. Stephen Thomas and Sandra Crouse Quinn, of the University of Maryland, identified a direct connection between the legacy of Tuskegee and the high degree of basic mistrust among African Americans toward the American biomedical establishment. In a survey on attitudes toward AIDS among members of that community done in 1990 by the Southern Christian Leadership Conference, 35 percent of the respondents stated that they viewed AIDS as a form of genocide, and 44 percent that they believed that the government was "not telling the truth" about AIDS. Separately, Harlon Dalton, a professor of law at Yale University and a member of the National Commission on AIDS, cited the legacy of Tuskegee in his 1988 essay "AIDS in Blackface" as one of the reasons for the African

American community's reluctance "to 'own' the AIDS epidemic": "It is a predictable outgrowth of the problematic relationship between the black community and the larger society, a relationship characterized by domination and subordination, mutual fear and mutual disrespect, a sense of otherness and a pervasive neglect that rarely feels benign."[57]

Physicians have often felt torn between what they perceive as their dual loyalty toward their patients and toward society. The obligation of physicians to their patients is (or should be) a given, based upon codes of physician conduct extending at least as far back as the days of Hippocrates, codes that enshrine physicians' responsibilities toward their patients. However, with the adoption of third-party payment systems for health-care expenses (including physician fees) by governments and health insurance companies—and the increased regulatory oversight that has accompanied this—physicians truly have become the servants of two masters. In this case, he who pays the piper often calls the tune.

HOW INTRUSIONS BY THIRD-PARTIES INTERFERE WITH PHYSICIAN-PATIENT COMMUNICATION

The implications for the physician-patient relationship when a third party (government, society, or payor) has a seat at the table cannot be overstated. The third party does not always directly interact with the patient, leaving her in many cases oblivious to the powerful influence it exerts over the physician with all that relates to treatment options and preference and how these are presented to—or hidden from—the patient. The end result, however, is that the physician ceases to be solely committed to the patient's well-being and to working toward bringing the patient to the best possible health outcomes. This conflict of interest is obvious when the third-party pressures physicians to choose less expensive but perhaps less effective treatments in order to save money. Because the third party may actually be the one paying the physician, it is able to reward or to punish him, depending upon how closely he upholds its mandates. When the third party is the government, it may also use its legislative authority to determine what the physician may or may not offer or discuss with patients. This, too, undermines the trust patients have in their physicians. How could you possibly trust your doctor to look out for your own best interests knowing that she was ordering unnecessary testing—or actually forbidden from discussing the very reasons your health was being compromised?

In the United States, there has been a recent flurry of legislation regulating medical practice and communication between physician and patient that has everything to do about politics and nothing to do with either medicine or good patient care. The American College of Physicians (ACP) has come out strongly against the growing trend of governmental interference in the physician-patient relationship, and in July 2012 released its "Statement of Principles on the Role of Governments in Regulating the Patient-Physician Relationship,"[58] which documented multiple examples of this phenomenon, including:

- Mandating that physicians inform women undergoing mammography of additional breast cancer screening options (Connecticut, Texas, and Virginia), even though these may not be suitable for all women and may in fact result in false-positive results, leading to unnecessary morbidity and mortality from additional testing
- Requiring the performance of medical testing such as ultrasound (Arizona, Virginia) prior to abortion, even though it is of no proven value in medical decision making for those situations. In Virginia the original bill would have required transvaginal ultrasound; the final version was modified after public outcry
- Forbidding physicians from discussing certain topics altogether with patients. This includes the counseling of patients about gun safety (Florida) and discussing the potential health risks from exposure to chemicals used in fracking (Pennsylvania)

Jeremy A. Lazarus, MD, president of the American Medical Association, has argued that "the ability of patients and physicians to have open and confidential conversations has always been the cornerstone of a successful health-care system. Lawmakers should not dictate the use of certain medical practices, nor should they threaten the open communication between physician and patient."[59]

Similarly, efforts to control health-care costs through managed care and capitation in the 1990s, in which patients' choice of physicians was limited and physicians and hospitals were provided financial incentives to reduce costs by eliminating unnecessary medical procedures and testing, led to significant public backlash. In an article for the *New York Times*, Erik Eckholm spoke with William Andereck, a Californian internist highly critical of these incentives:

> "'For the black and white stuff, [physicians] still make the same calls. But most of medicine isn't black and white. It's judgment calls, and that's where the incentive system has its impact.' If a woman has a lump in her breast, the doctor can wait three weeks or send her to the surgeon down the hall for an immediate biopsy, he noted. 'Probably the outcome will be the same,' he said. But over that three weeks, what if it was your wife?'"[60]

Some physician contracts with managed-care organizations in the 1990s forbade physicians from discussing with their patients medical services that were not covered by the patients' specific plans. This seriously undermined patient trust in their physicians, and, in general, patient trust in physicians is higher when the latter are paid through a fee-for-service model rather than one of managed care. This was also reflected in physician descriptions of the impact of managed care upon their practice. In one study in which more than one thousand primary-care physicians were surveyed, 65 percent described managed care as having had a negative effect on the overall primary care physician-patient relationship. Fifty-three percent of the physicians felt that their ability to place patients' best interests first was adversely affected by managed care. Two-thirds agreed that making the physician serve as a gatekeeper to prevent the overutilization of medical resources made him appear adversarial to patients.[61]

Some of these same concerns have been expressed about certain provisions in the Patient Protection and Affordable Care Act (PPACA, also known as Obamacare), specifically the establishment of the Patient Centered Outcomes Research Institute and the Independent Payment Advisory Board.[62] As John O'Shea wrote in his critique of similar provisions contained in H.R. 3200, America's Affordable Health Choices Act of 2009 (an earlier version of PPACA):

> Physicians understand the potential value of clinical care guidelines and even comparative effectiveness research as tools that can add to the fund of knowledge to help inform patients and physicians. But the ultimate decision regarding what is appropriate in an individual clinical situation should not be mandated or coerced by [Medicare Payment Advisory Commission], a health care czar, or any other "independent" entity.[63]

This is extremely important when considering what the role of government should be in reducing health-care expenses and what kind of effect that role may have on physician autonomy. It is especially important when legislation is proposed or enacted that mandates and/or proscribes actions on the part of physicians and limits their interactions with patients in ways that usurp medical decision making from physicians. Doing so enshrines into law the very dangerous principle that physicians' first loyalty is to the government and its political agenda and not to the patient.

In addition to the government and other third-party payors, other parties are often "present" at the meeting between physician and patient, specifically pharmaceutical and medical-device companies. Although they do not wield the same power that payors or governmental agencies do, they too can seriously undermine the trust between patient and physician. Instead of actually being seated at the table, they may stand off to the side, figuratively whispering in the physician's ear while remaining mostly invisible to the patient. The pharmaceutical and medical-device companies try to convince physicians to choose one medication or medical device over another, often via financial incentive. The historically overly close relationship between Big Pharma and physicians has made many on either side of the physician-patient divide uneasy.

A 2012 study found that a majority of patients were interested in knowing whether their physician accepted gifts from the pharmaceutical industry. Fifty-nine percent of patients stated that were that to be the case, their trust in that particular physician would be diminished. One quarter said that if they learned that their physician had received a gift in exchange for being briefed about a specific drug by a pharmaceutical company representative, they would be less inclined to take it. These findings are similar to those of earlier studies which also, unsurprisingly, showed a higher degree of acceptance by physicians, as compared with patients, of physicians receiving gifts or payments from the pharmaceutical industry. However, even though physicians as a group seem more accepting of this practice, with many professing not to be influenced by the gifts they receive, this acceptance does not always translate into a willingness to publicly disclose their financial ties with the pharmaceutical industry. According to one recent study, more than 35 percent of physicians disagreed with the need to make their patients aware of any financial relationships that they maintained with either drug companies or medical-device manufacturers.[64]

This is a problem, as there is a robust body of evidence to justify the cynicism expressed by patients toward physicians who receive gifts from pharmaceutical companies and how these gifts influence medical decision making. Physicians who receive gifts from pharmaceutical representatives tend to have more positive attitudes toward meeting with the representatives and also to believe that these meetings do not influence their prescription behavior—even though they do, in fact, make them more likely to prescribe the representatives' product.[65] The implication is clear: the industry provides gifts to disarm physicians of their suspicions and to get their reps through the office door; once inside, their goal of getting the physician to increase his use of their product will be achieved. This is consistent with human nature from time immemorial; in this modern-day version, the reps' suitcase loaded with freebies is a stand-in for the wooden horse used so effectively by Odysseus to seduce Troy's defenders into admitting his soldiers into the city.

The Physician Payments Sunshine Provisions of PPACA (Obamacare), which came into effect in 2013,[66] mandate reporting by the pharmaceutical and medical-device industries of all gifts to physicians and teaching hospitals valued at greater than ten dollars per recipient (or one hundred dollars in the aggregate). This provision has been criticized by some, including Thomas Stossel of Harvard Medical School, who in a sharply critical opinion piece in the *Wall Street Journal* decried the Sunshine Provisions as "a toxic rule" and advocated that Congress eliminate them before "they burn us [physicians and patients] all."[67] However, one may hope that the increased transparency about the ties between some physicians and the pharmaceutical industry will help diffuse some of the mistrust that has developed toward the medical profession as a whole among certain segments of the public.

CLOSING THOUGHTS

In this chapter, I've described how the patient's understanding of his disease, shaped both by personal experience and cultural background, can profoundly influence his illness behavior and how without understanding these it becomes very difficult for the physician to draw upon or to modify them so as to bring about the desired outcomes. Likewise, the "sick role" cast upon patients by society not only influences illness behavior in the patient but the physician's behavior as well, even when she is unaware of its influence. In the next chapter, I'll provide examples of the difference between treating disease and treating disease *and* illness, discuss the importance of doing both, and demonstrate how central good communication between physician and patient is to making such a thing possible.

5

BODY AND SOUL

A **FEW MONTHS** after starting my pediatrics residency in Israel, a three-month-old baby boy named Tomer was admitted to our department because of the onset of seizures. However, it was clear that there was much more going on with him as well. Although still very young, we could see that he was already developmentally delayed. His muscle tone was lower than would have been expected for someone his age, he didn't maintain eye contact, and he had not yet begun to smile.

Based upon the chief resident's previous experience with other babies who'd presented like this in the past, he assumed that Tomer would become a regular patient of ours. He asked me to become Tomer's primary pediatrician within our department, explaining that it would be best for the family and child to have one person who would really know him and be able to maintain continuity of care for what would likely become an extended relationship. He also said that he thought that I'd learn a lot from caring for Tomer. I agreed, even though assuming overall responsibility for this particular child's care made me quite anxious. I myself had a healthy two-month-old son at home, and while they were already so different, I couldn't help but compare them and wonder whether my own son, Yuval, might also start to seize one day, just as Tomer had. However, I was able to suppress those fears and by the next day felt entirely up to task.

And so began an intense relationship between Tomer, his parents, and me, a relationship that spanned the next five months of his life. Tomer, as we later found out, suffered from a rare and incurable metabolic disorder. Powerless to halt the relentless progression of his disease, we were able only to treat his symptoms as his different organ systems began to shut down, one after the other.

On balance, Tomer spent more time in the hospital than at home during those months, just as my chief resident had predicted. Sometimes Tomer would arrive after an especially prolonged seizure, almost comatose from all of the meds he'd been given during the ambulance ride over in an attempt to break the seizure, and would stay with us for a few hours until their effects had worn off and he was safe to go home. On other occasions, he'd be admitted for several days. With each admission, Tomer seemed to have regressed further and to have become weaker and less interactive than before.

It was especially cold and wet on the night that Tomer died. He had already been admitted for a couple of weeks by then, and over the preceding days Tomer's breathing pattern had become irregular. The pauses in his breathing had become longer and more frequent, an ominous sign that the portion of his brainstem that controlled his breathing was no longer functioning properly. I was on call with Sigal, who was also well acquainted with Tomer and his parents. Sigal was a year ahead of me in her training and was covering the ICU that night.

I asked Sigal what I should do if Tomer were to die that night, as I had never before experienced that with a child whom I had cared for so closely. Sigal told me that the most important thing was to be present with, and for, the family. I had no clue what she meant by that, but Sigal reassured me that she'd be there for me and encouraged me to page her whenever I needed her.

A few minutes before midnight, I got paged out of the emergency room by Ina, the nurse caring for Tomer, because she and his parents had needed to use a bag and mask to resuscitate him numerous times over the preceding fifteen minutes. A new pattern had begun to set in. Tomer would stop breathing, his heart rate would fall, and they'd give him several breaths with the bag and mask. He'd come back up for a short while, but after several seconds would once again stop breathing.

Tomer's family and I had had many conversations during the preceding month about what they would want us to do if and when he were no longer able to breathe on his own. His parents had been very clear about not wanting Tomer to be intubated or mechanically ventilated once that moment arrived. It had seemed very straightforward when discussed abstractly, yet now that he was actively dying, I was very unsure of what to do in the absence of any clearly defined plan.

Joined by Sigal, I went to Tomer's room. From the doorway, I could see Ina resuscitating Tomer with the bag and mask. Ina stopped when she noticed us. A few seconds later, the alarm from the monitor above his bed began to sound, indicating that once again, Tomer's heart rate was dropping.

Tomer's father, who was standing on the other side of the crib with his arms resting on the lowered railing, looked at me helplessly. He didn't say a word. Tomer's mother was seated on the low foldout bed, staring absently out the rain-splattered window into the darkness beyond. I just stood there, unable to move.

Entering the room, Sigal walked slowly over to Tomer's crib and stood next to his father. She stroked Tomer's face softly and looked up at the monitor screen. She turned to his father, and then to his mother, who had joined them at the crib side. Sigal put her arms around both parents' shoulders and drew them toward her.

"It's time," she whispered softly.

The father put his hand on Tomer's chest, while his mother shuddered silently, arms folded over her chest, tears streaming down her face. Sigal suggested that they say their final goodbyes to their son. Sigal, Ina, and I then left the room, closed the door behind us, and waited in silence outside.

Several minutes later the door opened and the parents stepped into the hallway. They were tearful and clearly distraught, but they also had a certain inner peace I'd not seen since we'd first met.

"Thank you," they said to us, and we embraced, somewhat stiffly. They left for home a short while later, and Sigal and I returned to work, a busy night awaiting both of us.

During the preceding months, I had come to know the whole family well, to the point where it seemed as though I had spent almost as much time with them as I had with my own wife and son. I felt awful for everything they had been through and more than anything wanted to be able to comfort them at that moment. Yet once Tomer was actually dying that evening, I realized that I was simply unable to connect with them emotionally. It was as if a part of me was completely frozen.

I became aware, suddenly, of just how poorly I actually *had* connected with Tomer's parents and how little I had allowed myself really to understand what it was that they had been feeling and struggling with, not just that night but during the entire time I'd been caring for him. I saw just how much I'd restricted my interactions with them to the professional aspects of treating his disease, at the exclusion of his illness, which had manifested mostly through his parents. Although our interactions had always been friendly, I had never really considered how their son's illness was affecting *them* or what their own emotional needs might be. This meant that once the focus of caring for Tomer had shifted completely away from him to his parents—whose needs had always been there, though I hadn't ever recognized them—I was completely at a loss for what to do.

It still amazes me that I was able to care so closely for Tomer, for so many months, without ever really connecting with his parents— and without even realizing that this connection was absent. Looking back from a distance of seventeen years, I can identify some mitigating explanations (perhaps). I had only just started my residency, with its intense schedule and demands, and had very little practical experience to draw upon. This required me to focus my attention on those things that seemed most important, namely, learning how to care for acutely sick kids and to keep them from dying. Caring for their parents seemed almost a luxury, certainly something of secondary importance. Additionally, walling off my emotions had been a useful defense mechanism for me; this had enabled me to care for Tomer without dwelling on how easily he could have been my own son. This kept my own anxieties in check. However, once Tomer began actively to die that night, my medical skills became superfluous. It was emotional support that his parents needed, and, thankfully, Sigal was there for them. I was ashamed at my inability to connect with Tomer's parents. It left me feeling utterly deficient at the time, and it continued to trouble me for years to come.

BEING PRESENT

Learning to be present with patients and their families, as Sigal had counseled me that night, is a process that can take years. It certainly took me that long. To me, at this stage of my life and career, being present means being sensitive and relating to not only my patients' disease but also to the illness and sickness that disease creates and that ripple outward to affect others, myself included. Recognizing all of these is part of being present.

For me, being present means listening and responding nonjudgmentally to what my patients and their family members say, verbally and nonverbally, with honesty, compassion, and empathy. It means avoiding platitude and cliché and allowing myself to be led by a natural curiosity about my patients and their families and what they are going through so that I can better understand their needs and do a better job of helping them. Once again, much of this extends far beyond the narrow definitions of disease. Being present means engaging with my patients and their families as a fellow human being who is also a physician rather than as someone trying to act out someone else's preconceived role of what a physician is supposed to do or to say.

Although I no longer actively have to remind myself to be present with my patients, I still have much to improve upon. Learning how to do this has, I think, been the most difficult part of my journey to become a good healer. I do believe, however, that it has also been the most important part and certainly the most rewarding.

A couple of years later, I had another opportunity to observe from up close what being present actually meant. This time, I was able to recognize it for what it was.

The morning that Batya died was also the first time that I ever personally took care of her. I had only just returned to the department after spending six months working on a basic-science research project in a lab at another hospital. Although Batya had been a patient in the department on several of my call shifts during that period, and I had heard her discussed many times at morning report and at other departmental meetings, my interactions with her family had been very limited. I don't think that we had ever exchanged more than a few words until that day.

Batya was six months old. Soon after she was born, she was diagnosed with type-one spinal muscular atrophy (SMA-1), a rare neuromuscular disease that causes profound and progressive muscle weakness. Most infants who are born with SMA-1 die before their first birthday, usually because of respiratory failure.

Batya had been admitted multiple times because of complications arising from her increasing difficulties with breathing and feeding. It was clear to everyone in the department that her condition was deteriorating, and many of the senior physicians had told Batya's mother that her daughter's prognosis was very poor. The family's pediatrician, too, had conveyed the same message many times. Yet Batya's mother seemed neither to hear nor to accept what she was being told as far as her daughter's prognosis was concerned. Batya's health would fail, and her mother would bring her in to the emergency room. There Batya would be stabilized, start treatment for the aspiration pneumonia that was almost always the cause of her distress, and be admitted. A few days later, Batya would be sent home, only to return shortly thereafter because of another life-threatening event.

I was working in the emergency room that morning when Batya was brought in by two medics, her mother following right behind them. One of the medics was ventilating Batya with a bag and mask; the other carried a portable tank of oxygen connected to the bag by a thin, transparent tube. Batya's eyes were closed, and her color was ashen. A few hours earlier, we learned, Batya had developed what initially appeared to be just minor nasal congestion, but this soon snowballed into respiratory distress that rapidly overwhelmed her. The medics had tried to intubate her on their way to the hospital but were unsuccessful. Instead, they wound up bagging her with oxygen during the twenty-minute ride.

The medic gently rested Batya on the crash bed, and one of the nurses connected her to the monitor. Pausing the bagging for about twenty seconds so that we could get a sense of how serious her condition was, we watched as her heart rate plummeted into the low thirties. Her breathing was agonal. The isolated and irregular gasps she drew were insufficient to survive. Without additional assistance, she would die.

Had this been any other kid, she would have been well on her way to being intubated and on a ventilator. But everyone in the department who knew her, or of her, understood that Batya's condition was terminal. This is, unfortunately, how babies with SMA-1 often die. It seemed futile to push forward with a full-blown resuscitation. However, the other resident working with me that morning, Ronit, had also just returned from an extended period away from the department and she, too, had had no previous interaction with either Batya or her mother.

Because neither of us had an existing relationship with the family, we felt uncomfortable at that moment discussing with the mother whether or not to proceed with resuscitation. It seemed inappropriate for either Ronit or me to put the mother on the spot like that and to ask her whether we should let her child die peacefully instead of proceeding down the path of aggressive intervention. Yet we also felt that going forward with a full-blown resuscitation would be not only futile but wrong and that it would subject Batya to significant discomfort while serving only to postpone the inevitable by hours or days. Our unease was only made more acute by Batya's mother's silence. She stood there at the bedside, silently stroking her daughter's foot, eyes glued to the monitor, saying nothing. Absolutely nothing.

Ronit put the mask back over Batya's face and resumed bagging. Batya's heart rate picked back up again, but aside from the rapid blips on the monitor, we could discern no other signs of life. Except for the rise of her chest each time Ronit squeezed the bag, Batya lay motionless.

We looked at each other, both thinking the same thing. I asked one of the nurses if the attending who was supposed to be with us in the ER that morning had returned from the meeting he had gone to, hoping that he would call the code, stop the resuscitation efforts, and allow Batya to die in peace. Unfortunately, he was nowhere to be found.

I'm not sure how my department chief learned about what was going on, but suddenly, there she was, standing next to Batya's mother. Wordlessly, she put her arm around the mother's shoulders and drew Batya's mother toward her.

"I'm so sorry," Dr. Sinai said softly.

All at once, the tension seemed to evaporate from the mother's body. She began to sob, burying her head in Dr. Sinai's chest as she embraced her with both arms. Ronit slowly put the mask and bag down on the bed. A few seconds later, I reached over and turned off the monitor. Then, I shut off the oxygen.

No one said anything.

After about a minute, Dr. Sinai and the mother left the room and slowly walked over to Dr. Sinai's office, arms on each other's shoulders, Batya's mother's head on Dr. Sinai's chest. A few minutes later, Ronit and I pronounced Batya dead.

Levana Sinai, the chief of the pediatrics department where I did my residency, was one of my most influential teachers and role models. Some of the residents liked her more than others—I personally thought she was amazing—but we all had nothing but the highest respect for her. Possessing incredible clinical skills, she demanded excellence from each and every one of us. Nothing less than that would do, ever. She could be intimidating, even fearsome at times. The last thing any of us ever wanted to do was to disappoint her. Her intolerance of anyone foolish enough to try to cut corners with patients was as legendary as it was unforgiving.

None of her toughness was on display that morning, however. Instead, what I saw were her compassion and empathy. With those three words, "I'm so sorry," and even more so, with her embrace, silences, and presence, she succeeded in connecting with Batya's mother so much more than either Ronit or I could have and in bringing an unbearable situation to its best possible conclusion.

Because Dr. Sinai had already established a relationship with Batya's mother and was attuned to and understood her complex and often contradictory feelings about caring for a terminally ill child—and above all, by being simply herself—Dr. Sinai was able to help this mother through this most difficult of moments. Once again, I was amazed at the powerful effect being present with a patient and her family could have, just as I had observed with Sigal two years earlier.

COMMUNICATION-SKILLS TRAINING

Beyond a physician's knowledge-based capabilities, the ability to be present is only one of the many emotional and spiritual skills that are necessary for her to reach her full healing potential. Compassion, empathy, integrity, and respect—these are also vitally important. Not everyone, however, enters or graduates from medical school with these attributes fully developed or with the ability to access them naturally, as I discovered the night Tomer died. This is where communication-skills training can be very helpful. Teaching medical students, interns, residents, and fully trained physicians to pay attention to the details of their interactions with patients can help them improve their quality, resulting in all of the benefits mentioned throughout this book. Communication-skills training also, unsurprisingly, leads to greater patient involvement during clinical visits and in their overall care, which, as will be discussed in chapter 7, is associated with both better health outcomes and lower health-care costs. Recognizing this, communication and interpersonal-skills training has been one of the six core competencies that the Accreditation Council for Graduate

Medical Education has required be addressed during residency training since 1999, though the degree to which this is carried out, and the aspects of each that are emphasized, vary widely between programs and specialties.[1]

Effective communication-skills teaching may involve lectures about the use of body language (maintaining eye contact, leaning forward while listening), or the use of computer-based teaching modules that focus on improving communication skills and empathy. It may also involve role-reversal training sessions, in which medical students assume the roles of patients in order to experience at first hand what it is like to struggle with communication barriers that interfere with access to health care. Likewise, workshops for medical residents that focus on specific weaknesses in physician-patient communication can yield long-term improvements in self-reported behavior. This includes, for example, learning how to become more proficient at gauging medication adherence or becoming more skilled at teaching patients how to take their medications properly. The use of personal coaches to teach experienced physicians how better to communicate with their patients has also been found to improve patient satisfaction, an indirect though important measure of success.[2]

Experiential simulation workshops are an excellent way of improving physician communication and relational skills. These typically involve role-playing by facilitators and participants or the use of standardized patients.[3] One especially effective educational approach is the Program to Enhance Relational and Communication Skills (PERCS) workshops, offered by the Institute for Professionalism and Ethical Practice (IPEP) at Boston Children's Hospital. PERCS involves using professional actors to play the roles of patients and their parents in a variety of realistic clinical scenarios. These workshops are interprofessional in nature, not geared exclusively to physicians, and are typically attended by nurses, chaplains, medical interpreters, respiratory therapists, social workers, psychologists, and child life specialists.

Another important feature of the PERCS workshops is the involvement of family-faculty members who contribute to the case scenarios, curriculum development, and teaching.[4] In the scenarios, the workshop participants interact in their typical clinical roles with the professional actors. For example, physicians take on the role of a physician (though not necessarily at their own level of training), and the same is true for the other health-care professional participants. The scenarios are conducted in simulated clinical environments that are physically very similar to those in which they might typically occur. For example, a conversation about the withdrawal of life support from a child who has suffered irreversible neurological devastation takes place in a room that is identical in design and layout to one of the meeting rooms in the hospital's intensive-care unit. The room is wired for audio and video, which are streamed back to the main meeting room where the other participants in the workshop can observe the conversations in real time as they are taking place. Although everyone participating is aware that these are only simulations, they feel very real both to participants and observers.

Having participated in a number of these workshops as well as having led similar ones for pediatric-pulmonary trainees, it is clear to me that the decision by IPEP to work with professional actors—which I had no part in—was a brilliant one. The actors' feedback is invaluable. They don't just portray the parent or patient: they *transform* themselves into the roles they assume. Full-time students of human behavior, the improvisational actors are able to pick up on nuances in the words and body language of the participants that might easily escape others. The actors spontaneously and seamlessly draw upon and respond to the cues of the participants as the scenarios unfold, and no two enactments are ever precisely the same.

Immediately following the simulations, which typically last between ten and fifteen minutes, all of the participants, including the actors, return to the main classroom for debriefing. During the debriefings, which are conducted by interdisciplinary faculty with appreciative inquiry, both the participants and actors are able to describe eloquently and in great detail what did and what did not work in the simulated encounter they have just experienced together.

Participants in these PERCS workshops have reported sustained improvements in their communication and relational skills as well as enhanced awareness of the perspectives of families struggling with having an acutely ill child. This has also been reported for other, similarly constructed workshops done elsewhere.[5]

During the last few years my colleagues and I have led other, similar simulation workshops for trainees in pediatric pulmonology, which include scenarios in which difficult conversations take place. As in the PERCS simulations, professional actors act out the roles of parents of very sick children, and the trainees play themselves, but with one major difference: there is no attending physician present to intercede if and when things get dicey, as there would otherwise be under normal circumstances.

In some of the scenarios we ask the actors playing the role of the parents of a seriously ill child who is more than likely to make a full recovery to inquire about their child's prognosis. It is striking to observe the difficulty some of the trainees have in telling the parents that they think that the child is going to be fine, rather than hedging and giving what they see as a more neutral "role-appropriate" response. For example, instead of reassuring the parents that the child will almost certainly be going home in two or three days, they will often offer up a boilerplate response full of guarded prognostications couched in potential complications, none of which is especially likely to occur.

During the debriefings which follow, I usually ask the trainees why they were so hesitant to offer more encouragement to the parents based upon their own experience. They often explain that they felt that they needed to be cautious about committing to the child making a full recovery, which they couldn't guarantee, after all, even though it was the most likely outcome. When I ask, however, what they think the likely outcome would have been, they invariably tell me that they are confident that the kid would have been just fine.

I know that that's not what I'd want from my own physicians if I were a patient. The whole purpose of consulting with physicians is to draw upon their years of experience and first-hand observation as well as what they've learned from the collective experience of other physicians. Unless these are freely shared, the patient is placed at a serious disadvantage and left unable to make informed choices and decisions about his care. This can generate a lot of unnecessary stress, something that emerges quite often in these simulation enactments.

This is certainly not what most patients and their families want, either. As a second-year pediatric resident doing a six-month rotation in the neonatal intensive-care unit (NICU) in Rehovot, I struggled with these very same issues myself. Somehow, somewhere, it had been drilled into my head that making positive assessments that could not be backed up with solid supportive evidence was tantamount to inviting a malpractice suit if and when they did not materialize. One day, one of my attendings overheard me hedging on the prognosis of one of the preemies in the NICU, who had had a very uneventful course in the unit and was going to be sent home within a few days. His mother had asked me whether her infant would grow up to be a "normal" child. He had been born relatively late in his gestation compared to many of the other kids we cared for, had had no brain bleeds, and really had required very little support or assistance during his stay. Still, I found it very difficult to answer her, both because of my relative inexperience as well as because of this nagging fear of committing to something over which I ultimately had no control. I gave the mother an evasive answer, something along the lines of "it's too soon to tell, we'll need to follow closely," etc.

Dr. Orna Flidel, who was my attending that month and had overheard our conversation, pulled me aside afterward and said that she felt that there was no reason I couldn't have put a more positive spin on my response, even without lying or making promises I couldn't keep.

"You could have told her that her baby has done extremely well so far, with none of the complications we often witness, and that you can see no reason why he shouldn't develop normally, though of course only time will tell. She *knows* you can't predict the future; what she was asking you was whether *you* think it is reasonable to even hope for a healthy baby. And in this case, it certainly is."

Orna then told me that several years earlier, she had been walking in downtown Rehovot when a woman approached her, called her by name, and hugged her.

"You may not remember me," she said, "but you cared for my Avivit just after she was born five years ago." The woman then put her hands on the shoulders of the girl standing next to her. Beaming, she turned her daughter slightly and shooed a stray wisp of hair from her forehead, showing her off to Orna.

"I am so grateful to you, Dr. Flidel," she continued. "Everyone else in the NICU told me she wouldn't make it. You were the only one who gave me hope, and look at her now!" she exclaimed.

Orna told me that the child was beautiful, an adorable kindergartener no different than any other. "It took a few seconds, but then it all came back to me. I had just come back to the NICU from my fellowship abroad when that baby was born. She had been very sick initially and developed early sepsis. No one knew if she'd survive, but there was something which made me feel she'd be OK, and I told the mother that, even though everyone else was painting a grim picture for her. We treated her aggressively, and she came through, very nicely, it turns out."

"And if you had thought she wouldn't make it?" I asked. "Would you have told her that as well?"

"Of course!" she responded, recoiling as if I'd just accused her of something horrible. "You *always* have to tell the truth, but the truth also includes how you see the patient's condition, even if your assessment is constantly in flux. That's what people are asking for. No one thinks you're promising them anything."

Orna paused. "Don't worry, Dennis, no one is going to mistake you for God!"

She laughed, and then grew serious again. "That is, as long as you don't pretend to *be* God. It's when doctors lose their humility that they get into trouble."

One of my colleagues at Boston Children's Hospital, Peter Weinstock, is an attending physician in one of the intensive-care units. He describes one of his roles when taking care of extremely sick children to me as serving as "the barometer of the parent's anxiety." By this he means that he tries to guide the patient's family hopes and fears in the direction he sees that things are heading. Ultimately, far more important to parents than the specifics of test results or imaging studies are whether or not their child will survive and in what condition he or she is likely to emerge. And these were exactly the questions that Orna had answered for Avivit's mother. By doing so, she had helped allay the mother's fears and had enabled the mother to place her child's condition within a context that she could relate to more easily than the dry specifics of her daughter's blood cultures or the daily changes being made to her ventilator.

BREAKING BAD NEWS

I was two weeks into an elective rotation at a pediatric ward in a small Israeli hospital located far from any major city. It was my final year of medical school, and we had just admitted a three-year-old child because of several days of fever, increasing pallor, and widespread bruising. On examination we discovered that his spleen, usually hidden beneath the ribs and quite difficult to palpate in young children, was significantly enlarged, extending almost to his belly button. He also had enlarged lymph nodes, easily felt all over his body. All of us were concerned that this child had more than just a routine, self-limited infection. We decided to schedule a bone-marrow biopsy for the next morning.

After the biopsy, I accompanied the pediatric oncologist to the pathology lab to look at the marrow slides. Under the microscope we could see that instead of containing the usual variety of different cell types, the boy's bone marrow had been taken over almost completely by what appeared to be sheets of large purple cells. These were immature lymphocytes, whose uncontrolled proliferation was, as we had suspected, the cause of the child's signs and symptoms. He had acute lymphoblastic leukemia. Once uniformly fatal, the prognosis for childhood leukemia has improved dramatically over the last decades, with survival from some forms topping 85 percent.[6] Even so, the reality is that many children do not survive the disease and/or its treatments, which are spread over many months and can be fraught with unpleasant side effects and complications.

Walking back from the lab, I asked the oncologist if I could be present when he met with the parents. "Of course," he replied. We stopped by the child's room and asked the child's parents to accompany us to the department chief's office to discuss the biopsy results.

The office was just down the hall from the child's room, and as we walked there I began to regret having asked to participate in the meeting. I was especially unsettled by the parents' demeanor, which seemed nonchalant in the extreme as they followed us down the corridor. It was excruciating to listen to them giggling and teasing each other, knowing as I did what terrible news awaited them. How was it even possible, I wondered, that they did not sense the gravity of their situation? Their son had just had a bone-marrow biopsy, after all. Although I had not been present when the procedure was discussed and consent obtained, I was certain that they had to have been told why it had been considered necessary.

After closing the door behind the parents, I sat down between them and the oncologist so that I would be able to observe all three simultaneously. The oncologist glanced down quickly at the printed pathology report in his hand, as if to reaffirm what we had just seen ourselves under the microscope, and then looked up at the parents. They were both still smiling and looked almost cheerful, as if they were expecting to find out which prize they had just won at a raffle.

"Your son has leukemia," the oncologist told them without any preamble. He then added, as if for emphasis: "blood cancer."

The parents responded as if they had just been physically struck; the change was instantaneous. The mother began to wail, and the father drew her toward him. After a few seconds, he looked up at the oncologist.

"Are you sure?" he asked.

Before the oncologist could answer, the mother cried out "He's going to die!" and collapsed, sobbing, into her husband's arms.

I was shocked at how badly this had unfolded. Surely, I thought, the news could have been broken to the parents in a better way. As the oncologist began to describe the different treatments and procedures that their child would need to undergo over the next several months, I could tell that the parents were absorbing nothing. Unable any longer to deny how serious their son's condition was, they were now completely overwhelmed.

"Shai needs me; I have to go," said the mother abruptly.

Standing up, she grabbed a sheet of paper towel from the dispenser next to the door and, after wiping the tears and snot from her face, strode out of the room. The father remained seated for a few moments longer, looking down at his shoes, and then he, too, got up and walked out of the room without a word, as if we were no longer there.

The oncologist, meanwhile, had turned away toward the window and was now gazing off into the distance at the trees swaying in the afternoon breeze. He seemed serene, almost unfazed by the parents' reaction. After several seconds, he turned to me and commented that in his experience, some parents take this kind of news harder than others but that their response was not especially unusual. The tone of his voice was detached and sounded not much different than if he'd been describing the weather.

He and I spoke for a few more minutes, and then I returned to the ward. It was in chaos. The family was already half out the door. The shock and grief that I'd seen only minutes before had been replaced by anger. The father was berating one of the residents in the middle of the hall, and heads were emerging from the different rooms as other parents tried to hear what all the commotion was all about.

"We're leaving," the father was shouting. "You people know nothing! You just want to experiment on my child," he continued, "and there's no way that I'll allow a bunch of ignorant charlatans such as you to take care of my son."

Less than ten minutes later they were gone. Later that afternoon, we received a call from a hospital in Tel Aviv with a request to forward them the child's medical records. Apparently, the family had driven straight there after leaving us.

I think it is fair to assume that had the oncologist done a better job of communicating the child's diagnosis to the parents, everything might have gone much differently. For weeks and months afterward, I replayed that conversation in my mind, trying to learn from it and resolving to keep it as a personal example of how not to communicate with patients and their families.

Even so, and despite my best efforts, I still get it wrong sometimes.

Seven years later, I was in the third month of my pediatric-pulmonology fellowship at Boston Children's Hospital. During the interval period I had completed my studies, an internship, a residency in pediatrics, and had also worked as an attending pediatrician. I felt good about my capabilities and saw myself as a seasoned and experienced clinician. During that particular week I was covering the pulmonary inpatient service, and most of our patients had cystic fibrosis (CF). Patients with CF who become infected with certain strains of bacteria can have a more rapid decline in their lung function than others who are not. This is the reason for the strict infection-control measures that are enforced to keep patients with CF from passing their germs on to one another.

Sally was a beautiful six-year-old redhead with CF who had just been admitted to our service that afternoon after being seen earlier in the week in the outpatient clinic because of increased cough, shortness of breath, and weight loss. Labs had been sent, the admission scheduled, and I was now on my way up to see Sally, to take a history and examine her, and to discuss the treatment plan with her and her mother.

As I read through Sally's chart, I learned that she had an older brother who also had CF and who was much sicker than she was. Although both siblings were infected with a bug called *pseudomonas*, there were differences in the sensitivities of their bacteria to various antibiotics, suggesting that each was colonized with a different strain. I also saw that her most recent throat culture was positive for one of the more virulent bugs that can colonize patients with CF, *burkholderia cepacia* (*cepacia* for short). Neither she nor her brother had ever grown cepacia before, and this particular bug was resistant to most antibiotics, as is often the case with cepacia. This meant that we would need to send off a sample to a lab that did specialized testing to identify particular combinations of antibiotics with a synergistic effect, in the hope that at least one might be found that might prove successful at beating the infection down.

I called my attending physician who, coincidentally, was also Sally's and her brother's primary pulmonologist, to ask whether the family knew that she had grown cepacia and to solicit advice about which antibiotics to start. He surprised me when he told me that he himself had not been aware of the results of the culture. Apparently, they had only just been released by the lab that day.

"What should I do?" I asked him.

"Just tell the family what the culture grew," he counseled, "and explain that we'll start antibiotics based upon her previous cultures until the results of the synergy testing come back in another few weeks."

That made sense, I thought, and went up to the floor to see Sally and her mother. This was my first time meeting them, and both were very pleasant. The mother was especially gracious toward me, seeming to recognize that I had only just begun my fellowship. Over the course of our conversation, Sally's mother told me how sick Sally's brother was and how grateful she was that neither of her children had become infected with cepacia, especially Sally's brother, whose condition she feared would rapidly deteriorate rapidly were this to happen.

And this is where I really messed up.

Identifying what appeared to be a good opportunity to tell Sally's mother about the results of her daughter's throat culture, I responded by saying something like: "Sally's most recent throat culture did, in fact, grow cepacia, but . . ."

Before I could say anything else, Sally's mother let out a shriek, clasped both hands to her cheeks, and ran out of the room.

"Ohmigod ohmigod ohmigod," I heard her crying out in the hallway, her voice muffled by the door and her tears.

As incredible as this may sound, I was completely surprised by her reaction. Although Sally's mother had just told me how thankful she was that neither of her children had been infected with cepacia, I had somehow not heard just how significant this new piece of information would be to her. Instead of listening to what she was telling me about what the *illness* of cepacia and the sick role it would entail would mean to her and her children, I was allowing myself to be guided in this interaction solely by my previous experiences with treating the *disease* of cepacia. I'd already had the opportunity to take care of a number of patients with cepacia since starting my fellowship. Some were doing better than others, but on the whole, I had gotten the sense that they and their families, as well as the senior pulmonologists, were more focused on the patients' overall condition than on the specific bugs they grew. And so, even though Sally's mother had been very clear about how ominously she would view the appearance of this new strain of bacteria, I simply hadn't listened to her.

I looked at Sally, who hadn't said a thing since her mother had run out of the room. She was sitting up cross-legged in bed, sucking on a lollypop. She eyed me reproachfully and then turned away toward the muted television screen, ignoring me completely.

I knew that I needed to resolve things with her mother, though I had no idea of what I might say or how I might even begin to defuse the situation. Stepping out into the hallway I met the charge nurse, who had already guided Sally's mother into the conference room where she continued to sob loudly. Together, the charge nurse and I went inside.

"I'm so sorry . . ." I began, as I sat down.

Sally's mother looked at me, blinked, stood up, and left the room. The charge nurse followed her, leaving me alone in the room and feeling just terrible. I began to question why I had ever come to Boston in the first place. Clearly, I wasn't cut out for this.

After a couple of minutes, Sally's mother returned with the charge nurse. This time, I waited in silence until she started talking. For the better part of the next thirty minutes, Sally's mother upbraided me for having been so heartless and inconsiderate in breaking the news of what she perceived as her daughter's death sentence in such a callous manner, and in front of Sally, no less! I apologized again and again. I felt awful.

In retrospect, I know that I should have done a much better job of informing Sally's mother about her daughter's new infection, and that if I had, our whole interaction would have gone much differently. Twelve years later, I see that by being so focused on caring for Sally's disease and the responsibilities that doing so imposed upon me, mostly in the realms of diagnosis and treatment, I had completely failed to consider those components of illness and sickness which were so important to Sally's mother. Even though I had five additional years of experience under my belt, I had still made the same mistake with Sally as I had with Tomer's parents at the beginning of my residency. By attending only to Sally's disease I was ignoring other needs that she, and especially her mother, had. Or as the psychiatrist George Engel might have described it: I was focusing solely on the *biomedical* at the expense of the *biopsychosocial* aspects of her disease, that is, her illness and sickness.[7] The medicine I was practicing was, at its foundation, unidirectional and impersonal, even though I earnestly aspired to be as compassionate toward Sally, her mother, and all of my patients as I could possibly be.

While the difference between treating *disease* and treating *disease*, *illness*, and *sickness* may sound like one solely of semantics, there is a world of difference between them. A physician who treats only disease is like an artist who concentrates on his technique so that his performance, taken in passively by the audience, will be the best it possibly can. However, the quality of his performance does not for the most part depend upon the particular audience members. Bruce Springsteen will give the same electrifying show regardless of whether you, or I, or neither one of us is there in the crowd to cheer him on. The practice of medicine that sets as its twin goals both physical *and* psychosocial healing is different, however. Unless the physician is attentive to the patient's illness and sickness experiences, and to what drives and accentuates them, they will remain neglected and the patient's broader needs left unsatisfied and unfulfilled.

RECOGNIZING AND WORKING AROUND DEFENSE MECHANISMS

Common to my interaction with Sally's mother and the oncologist's with Shai's parents was the abrupt shattering of the defense mechanisms that the parents had constructed to ward off the anxiety that their children's situations would otherwise have generated. Going into that fateful meeting, Shai's parents denied the very real possibility that he might have a life-threatening disease. Sally's mother, too, had invested an enormous amount of energy trying to protect her children from becoming infected with a bug that she was convinced would surely kill them. As long as they were free of cepacia, they were sick, but in ways she felt could be controlled (notwithstanding the fact that Sally's brother was already very sick even without it). Becoming a *CF patient with cepacia* was something Sally's mother had worked heroically at trying to prevent for either sibling—ultimately, to no avail. Upon learning that Sally had become infected despite her best efforts to prevent this from happening, it became abruptly clear to Sally's mother how little control she had over the course of their disease.

We all rely upon defense mechanisms to one degree or another to avoid becoming incapacitated by anxiety. Defense mechanisms can be very useful for dealing with abstract problems (rationalization: *I know that it's theoretically possible for the church to be struck by a meteorite while I'm getting married, but the statistical likelihood of that happening is very small, so I really don't need to worry about it too much*). They do not, however, actually solve the problems or make them go away. Instead, they provide a framework for resolving the anxiety that the problems generate, and because of this, they can sometimes become barriers to resolving the problems effectively (denial: *That lump in my breast which is getting bigger and beginning to ooze blood on my bra is probably just a really bad pimple*).

During my psychiatry clerkship at Hadassah hospital in Jerusalem, one of the psychiatrists cautioned me to remember that people construct and rely upon defense mechanisms for good reason. Dismantling them can have severe consequences, he warned me, and if and when you do decide to do so, he said, you'd better be prepared to deal with the consequences.

This is why one of the most effective ways of beginning a difficult conversation, whether including the sharing of bad news or the disclosure of a medical error or complication, involves asking the patient and/or the family to describe and explain what they understand about the current situation. This gives a sense of what the patient actually is or is not aware of regarding his condition and helps the physician avoid making unfounded assumptions. It can alert the physician to gaps in comprehension that need to be addressed at the onset, often very carefully, so as not to pull the proverbial rug out from under them as I did with Sally's mother. It also sheds light on how the patient is coping with the anxiety generated by the fact that the conversation even needs to take place.

In many cases, as the patient and/or family explain how they understand the patient's condition, the very concerns that had been hidden just out of view begin to emerge: *I'm hoping this is just a viral infection, but most kids with viruses don't undergo bone-marrow biopsies, do they? The fact that we're having a formal meeting like this probably means that something more serious is going on . . .* When patients and/or their family members describe what they know about their situation, the alert clinician is often able to pick up on these unstated fears and to address them in ways that avoid an abrupt dismantling of the defense mechanism(s) that they've carefully constructed in order to contain them.

It should not be understood to imply, however, that this approach always works. Sometimes the defense mechanism employed is so

strong as to deny footing to any other explanation within their consciousness for the patient's situation. *My son just has a bad cold, and
those bruises must have come from falling down in the playground while
I wasn't looking.* When I sense that this is the case, I will usually start
out by recapitulating the circumstances leading up to our conversation.
I will then preface the disclosure of the bad news itself by letting the
patient and/or the family know that I'm about to share some bad news
with them. At that point, I usually pause and give them several seconds
to digest that before proceeding with the actual disclosure.

Letting bad news sink in and be processed is vitally important.
Some physicians feel uncomfortable with silences and feel a need to
talk through them. Although I observe this more commonly with
less experienced physicians, I've also seen some very senior ones make
the same mistake. This is as true when the patient is a layperson as it
is when he has a medical background: the common denominator is
the stress that continues to build under the onslaught of information
and that is never given an opportunity to defuse. This, I believe, was
the main reasons that the oncologist's conversation with Shai's parents had gone so badly. Not only were the parents caught off guard by
learning that their son had leukemia, but they suddenly found themselves bombarded by abstract concepts, unfamiliar jargon, and statistics about treatments and prognoses. Their world had just been turned
upside down, and they now found themselves being told that their son
would need to undergo all kind of medical and surgical procedures
they'd never heard of before. Is it any surprise that they just shut down
and walked out?

CLOSING THOUGHTS

In this chapter, I've tried to show why it is so important that physicians
expand their clinical focus beyond the confines of disease to include
illness, sickness, and other aspects of the patients' response to disease.
I've also attempted to highlight the importance of physicians being

attentive to their *own* responses to the multilayered effects of these different factors on their patients, recognizing them, and drawing upon them, so that they are able to provide their patients with better and more comprehensive care. In the next chapter, I'll discuss how bias and stigma, which often go unrecognized by physicians, affect their ability to communicate with their patients and how difficult it is for the physician to recognize that, in many instances, what he says is altogether different from what the patient hears.

6

RECONCILING
DIFFERENT WORLDVIEWS

The plague of mankind is the fear and rejection of diversity: mono-theism, monarchy, monogamy and, in our age, monomedicine. The belief that there is only one right way to live, only one right way to regulate religious, political, sexual, medical affairs is the root cause of the greatest threat to man: members of his own species, bent on ensuring his salvation, security, and sanity.

—Thomas Szasz, American psychiatrist (1920–2012)

MUCH OF an experienced physician's diagnostic process relies upon *heuristics*, mental shortcuts used in decision making that are based upon experiential knowledge and developed over a lifetime, based both upon personal experience as well as on that of others. Heuristics predispose people toward certain options when presented with choices, and once entrenched they are difficult to avoid without conscious effort. In decision making, these shortcuts can be beneficial but also detrimental, leading to serious errors of judgment, especially when employed in circumstances outside one's usual frame of reference. For physicians, this can happen when dealing with unusual disease presentations and when interacting with people whose illness and life experiences and/ or cultural mores are so different from what they are accustomed to that their usual decision-making heuristics simply do not apply to the specific circumstances at hand. While physicians would ideally step outside their usual thought and decision-making processes, it is very challenging to do so when unaware that these even exist.

The anthropologist Janelle Taylor identified the *culture of medicine* as one of the main causes of the clash between Lia Lee's immigrant Hmong parents and her physicians as described in Ann Fadiman's *The Spirit Catches You and You Fall Down*. Taylor wrote that "Lia's demise turns out to be not so much a 'collision of two cultures,' as a tragic encounter between (Hmong) 'culture' and (U.S. medical) 'science.'"[1] Taylor identified a lack of self-awareness on the part of Lia's physicians to their even being constrained not just by the norms of their own society but also by those of the very culture of biomedicine. She termed this obliviousness of physicians to the culture of their own profession "Medicine's 'culture of no culture'" and wrote that "physicians' medical knowledge is no less cultural for being real, just as patients' lived experiences and perspectives are no less real for being cultural."[2]

For her part, Fadiman described the difficulty that many physicians have in coming to terms with having what they regard as unassailable scientific truth being seen by their patients as just one more worldview on equal footing with any number of others. Dan Murphy, one of the Family Practice residents at Merced Community Medical Center who cared for Lia Lee during her many hospital visits, explained to Fadiman why the interaction between Lia's parents and the medical team was often so tense:

> People in the early years of their medical careers have invested an incredible amount of time and energy and pain in their training, and they have been taught that what they've learned in medical school is the only legitimate way to approach health problems. I think that is why some young physicians go through the roof when . . . patients reject what we have to offer them, because it intimates that what Western medicine has to offer is not much.[3]

Towards the end of *The Spirit Catches You and You Fall Down*, Fadiman writes that

> Western medicine is one-sided. Physicians endure medical school and residency in order to acquire knowledge that their patients do

not have. Until the culture of medicine changes, it would be asking a lot of them to consider, much less adopt, the notion that . . . "Our view of reality is only a view, not reality itself."[4]

The psychiatrist Thomas Szasz wryly wrote that "formerly, when religion was strong and science weak, men mistook magic for medicine; now, when science is strong and religion weak, men mistake medicine for magic."[5] The ones most susceptible to conflate the two are those desperate for a cure for themselves or a loved one and those who secretly wish that they were indeed empowered with special powers with which they might be able to reverse the course of nature itself.

According to Melanie Tervalon, from Children's Hospital, Oakland, and Jann Murray-Garcia, from UCSF, in order for physicians to overcome their inherent bias favoring biomedicine over other healing belief-systems, they must undergo "a process which requires humility in how physicians bring into check the power imbalances that exist in the dynamics of physician-patient communication . . . [and] to develop and maintain mutually respectful and dynamic partnerships with communities on behalf of individual patients and communities."[6]

Perhaps the most fundamental truth about the practice of medicine is that *all* that physicians do is ultimately about the patient and not about themselves. Though this should be obvious, recognizing (and acting on) it requires an abundance of humility, which not all physicians possess. It also requires self-confidence, which can be lacking in younger physicians at the start of their careers who have often endured years of reproach as medical students, interns, or junior residents from others more senior to them. It takes years of practice, in both senses of the word, for physicians to develop a sufficient mastery of biomedicine and to feel confident in their instincts once these are based not just on book knowledge but more importantly on their own experiences and those of their colleagues and teachers. And then, unexpectedly, they can find their judgment being questioned once again, this time by a patient instead of by a snarky chief resident.

That the very people whose health the physician is trying so hard to improve are now trying to second-guess her can seem downright insulting. Some physicians may feel that by questioning their advice or treatment plans, a patient is actually raising doubts about their professional competence and ability, both big pieces of their identities and sense of self-worth, and this can be deeply threatening. It can provoke responses that range from passive-aggression (*this is the treatment, and if you don't want to take/do/go through with it, there's nothing more I can do for you*) to defensiveness and even outright hostility.

Although it may indeed be true that the patient is concerned about the physician's abilities, it is also quite possible that the questions represent something else entirely. For example, they may instead represent part of the process of negotiation and bargaining, the third of five stages of struggle with impending death (or in this case, a diagnosis which may lead to disability or death) defined by Elizabeth Kübler-Ross in *On Death and Dying*.[7] Or, even more likely: the patient may simply have heard of other treatment possibilities for his condition and, realizing he may only have one chance at a cure, wants to make sure it's the best possible one.

I wish I could claim that I have been, or am now, immune to the hubris I'm describing. Unfortunately, however, that would simply not be true. And from my own experience I know that, as with Icarus, false pride and unchecked confidence almost always augur a disastrous fall.

One night during the second year of my pediatrics residency in Israel, I was on call for both the emergency room and one of the pediatric wards. As always, we were busy, and I only realized that something was amiss when I looked up from the baby whose IV I had just finished placing and noticed the activity on the other side of the treatment room. Seconds before, the doors had flown open, and two burly-looking orthodox Jewish men, both volunteers with Magen David Adom (the Red Star of David, the Israeli equivalent of the Red Cross), were already in the process of transferring a thin, rather sheepish-looking teen from the gurney they'd brought him in on over to the crash bed. At first glance the boy looked fine, apart from his obvious embarrassment at being the cause of such a commotion.

"Are you the doctor in charge?" asked one of the volunteers, catching my eye. Without waiting for the answer, he proceeded to tell me the background story. This was a fourteen-year-old who lived on one of the *moshavim* (rural farming communities) outside of Rehovot. Being driven home from basketball practice by the brother of a friend, he had jumped out of the van as it neared his house without waiting for it to come to a full stop. He landed badly, slipped, and struck his head without losing consciousness. On the ambulance ride over, he had vomited once, which explained why he smelled so sour.

Other than a generalized ache on the right side of his head, the boy said he felt fine. I examined him, and everything seemed to be in order. His vital signs were stable, as confirmed by the steady, high-pitched beeping of the monitor he'd been connected to. He had a moderate-size bump on the right side of his head, as well as a scalp abrasion where he had landed, but no evidence of a depressed skull fracture. He was oriented to time and to place, his pupils were equal and responsive, and the rest of his neurological examination was unremarkable. I decided to admit him for overnight observation. Although he seemed fine, I was troubled by the mechanism of his injury and by the fact that he had vomited.

Nowadays it would be routine in cases such as this to get a CT scan of the head to rule out a head bleed, which can be life threatening. The skull is like a hard box, and when blood accumulates within it and has nowhere else to go, it can put pressure on the brain, causing damage or death. Some of the signs that this may be happening include vomiting and/or changes in blood pressure, heart rate, size of the pupils, and consciousness. At that time, however, head scans were not done in Israel as a matter of course for every patient who had sustained mild head trauma. If there were strong suspicions that a patient might be bleeding, we would certainly get one, but most of the time we would admit the child for observation and serial examinations across a twenty-four-hour period, with further evaluation, including head imaging, on an as-needed basis.

As I was finishing up writing the admission orders, the boy's mother arrived after having heard from a neighbor about what had happened to her son. In tears, she hugged him, her black eyeliner running down her cheeks in asymmetric rivulets. She then turned to me and grabbed my arm:

"Doctor, will he be OK? Does he need a CT scan?"

As calmly as I could, I told her that yes, he'd be fine, but that I'd like to keep him for observation to make sure no further testing or interventions were needed.

She picked up immediately on the inherent contradiction in what I had just said. If his condition was unconcerning enough as to not warrant a scan, why did I want to admit him? And if I wasn't sure that he did not, in fact, have a head bleed, why not just go ahead and get the scan?

"I really think it's unlikely that anything serious has happened to him, but I do think that we need to watch him for the next several hours to be sure. And yes, we could get a scan, but that would expose him to radiation that would be best avoided unless there's no other choice."

She wasn't convinced and told me so. And even though I tried not to let it show, I could feel her getting under my skin. Why was she arguing with me? She wasn't a physician! Why didn't she defer to my superior knowledge and experience? Admittedly, I'd only been a resident for a year and a half, but after having been on call between eight and ten times each month for the last eighteen months, I was already pretty confident in what I was doing.

"He'll be fine," I told her, looking her straight in the eye and trying hard not to blink. "I'll be here all night. If anything changes I'll reassess and see if we need to do anything differently. Right now, though, I don't think he needs a scan."

She didn't buy it.

When I went to check in on him in the ward an hour later, he looked great. His examination was stable, and he hadn't vomited again. In fact, he had just eaten a sandwich. Aside from his head still hurting a bit, he felt fine.

"He looks really good," I told his mother, "and I'm very pleased. Hopefully, the rest of his stay will be uneventful, and you'll be able to go home tomorrow afternoon."

That was when she made eye contact with me for the first time since I'd walked into her son's room several minutes earlier:

"Doctor, shouldn't we get a CT scan? I'm really worried that something bad is going to happen."

Swallowing hard, I told her it wasn't necessary and quickly left the room.

Two hours later the floor nurse caring for the boy asked me to come to see him because he'd vomited. Nothing else about him had changed, but then, just as I finished examining him, he vomited again. The way he did was unusual, different from the way kids with stomach bugs throw up, for example. There was no deep heaving or retching. It was more like a small hiccough, except that it ended with vomit spilling out of his mouth.

"You see!" cried his mother, "I *told* you he's not right! What are you waiting for? Why don't you order the CT scan already?"

At that moment, I *really* didn't like this woman. I didn't like the way she was pressuring me like that, didn't like the fact that she didn't trust me, didn't like the way she made me feel like a bumbler. I knew much more about medicine than she did. This was rapidly deteriorating into a battle of egos, and I'm amazed and thankful, more than fifteen years later, that I was able to recognize the situation for what it was. Grateful that I was able to step back, reassess, and make the correct decision. Yes, if I were right, getting a scan would expose the boy to unnecessary radiation, as well as waste resources. But if I were wrong, and if these strange episodes of vomiting were indeed caused by her son's brain being compressed by the blood slowly filling his skull, it could prove fatal to him. And I'd never forgive myself.

So I ordered a scan, got a colleague to cover my other patients, and took him down to Radiology.

It shouldn't be much of a surprise that the scan showed that the boy did, in fact, have a medium-size accumulation of blood in the subdural area (the space between the thick fibrous tissue that covers the brain and the brain itself). Within an hour, we had transferred him to a larger hospital in Tel Aviv, where a neurosurgeon drained the accumulating blood later that night and from which he was discharged home a few days later without any complications.

That everything ended well for this kid (and for me!) is a matter of luck, really. Had I not been able to pivot away from the negative dynamic that had developed between the mother and me and instead continued to insist instead that *I* was right because *I* was the infallible physician, the night might have culminated in tragedy. One very valuable lesson I learned from that experience is that although reaching a diagnosis is critical to being able to treat a patient, that diagnosis constantly needs to be reevaluated. Without reassessing whether or not the diagnosis is correct and instead remaining wedded to a paradigm because of reasons that aren't germane to the patient and his care, a physician runs the risk of veering dangerously off target. The words of William Osler, one of the fathers of modern medicine, are just as relevant today as they were over a century ago: "Listen to the patient, and he will tell you the diagnosis."[8] In this case, we were all fortunate that I could hear what the boy was telling me through his symptoms, even though I really wanted to prove to his mother that I knew better than she did.

THE EFFECTS OF BIAS AND STIGMA ON COMMUNICATION BETWEEN PHYSICIANS AND PATIENTS

Tenaciously adhering to preexisting paradigms that are (or become) unsuited to unfolding clinical circumstances is not the only way heuristics get physicians (and their patients) into trouble. Faulty medical decision making that is based at least in part upon simple bias is no less pervasive or dangerous. *Implicit* bias, of which the holder is unaware, and *explicit* bias, of which he is, can both influence what treatments the physician offers to which patients, with the result that some receive suboptimal care relative to others being treated for the same conditions by the same provider. This was demonstrated by a study that investigated the presence of implicit racial bias toward African American patients among 287 physicians from Atlanta and Boston. The researchers found that even though the physicians denied explicit racial bias toward their African American patients, implicit association testing revealed attitudes characterizing these patients as being "less cooperative with medical procedures, and in general." The stronger the implicit bias, the less likely physicians were to follow accepted treatment guidelines for prescribing thrombolytic medicine to African American patients presenting with symptoms of coronary-artery blockage than they were to prescribe it to white patients who presented with similar complaints.[9] While it is certainly possible that there may have been other reasons that influenced these physicians' decisions about what to prescribe their patients, it may well have been that the physicians gave up too soon and simply didn't try hard enough to convince their African American patients to agree to standard treatment for their condition because of their implicit assumption that they, the patients, wouldn't follow through anyway.

Although a physician may be unaware of his own implicit biases, these are often picked up on by his patients. Physicians, after all, are just as likely as others to externalize their biases in their interactions with patients, even if they try not to or are unaware of their existence. A recent survey of a group of Latina and African American breast cancer survivors revealed that more than a third believed that they had suffered discrimination because of their race or ethnicity and that this had affected the quality of their care.[10] To be sure, this finding raises an interesting question. It is certainly possible that the discrimination these women subjectively perceived was not objectively present but rather sensed because of previous experiences they had had with other health-care providers. Regardless, however, the fact that so many of these patients shared the perception of being discriminated against is troubling.

The specific disease that brings patients to seek care from the physician can itself be a source of negative physician bias through the larger context of sickness, as I discussed in chapter 4. Researchers who interviewed fifty HIV-positive male American military veterans about their perceptions of HIV stigma in the context of health care heard descriptions of both passive and active stigmatization directed at them by their physicians. The passive stigmatization was mostly expressed nonverbally through diminished eye contact, physical distance maintained, and vocal tone and inflection. The men felt that this conveyed "various forms of negative affect, including irritation or anger, nervousness, or fear at having to work with HIV-positive clientele." The active stigmatization included overt abusiveness and/or refusal to treat. One man described

> [an] encounter with a physician who sought him out one evening in his hospital room to seemingly taunt him for his diagnosis. He explained "this little, goofy, bearded guy, says: 'you know you gonna die.' And he was a physician. He said, 'Do you know what kinda AIDS you got?' I said, 'Yeah, I got the AIDS that you can't cure.' He said: 'well, you know you don't got long to live.'"[11]

Janni Kinsler of the David Geffen School of Medicine, UCLA, and colleagues, interviewed 223 patients with HIV of low socioeconomic status in Los Angeles County. They found that 26 percent reported that at least one health-care provider had seemed uncomfortable with them, treated them in an inferior manner, and/or preferred to avoid serving them altogether. More than twice as many of those who felt stigmatized also reported difficulties in accessing medical care in comparison to those who didn't. Kinsler concluded:

> Patients who perceive their health care providers as being uncomfortable with them or treating them in an inferior manner could greatly affect their use of needed medical services, including antiretroviral therapy. Thus stigma may be an important barrier to

maintaining the health and longevity of those living with HIV. . . . Negative experiences with providers may discourage patients from returning for follow-up medical appointments, and may affect future relationships with health care providers such as patient-provider communication and trust.[12]

Another cause of stigmatization is an underlying attribute, such as obesity, which can be unrelated to the reason that brings the patient to the physician in the first place. A recent meta-analysis of thirty studies relating to professional and/or patient experiences surrounding obesity found evidence in all of them that the patients' obesity impaired interactions with health-care providers and services. This directly affected the quality of their medical care. One study of a group of female hospital employees in Wisconsin revealed that those who were overweight or obese were almost four times as likely either to delay or cancel their physician appointments outright when compared to women of normal weight. Seventy-two percent of the women admitted that this was because of embarrassment about their weight.[13]

Other studies have found that stigma, such as that attached to obesity, leads to decreased utilization of preventive medical services. Pap-smear testing for cervical cancer and mammography screening for breast cancer are less likely to be done in overweight and obese women than in their normal-weight peers. Once again, this is likely the result of a sense of stigma. One study found that 36 percent of morbidly obese women had experienced disrespectful treatment or negative attitudes from health-care providers.[14]

David Katz, the director of the Yale Prevention Research Center, described this phenomenon after meeting a new patient in clinic, an obese woman who had avoided physicians after they had repeatedly treated her "not as a patient, but as a fat patient":

I met a woman who should have received medical attention for a variety of remediable issues, but who had not. I met a woman who should have had cancer screening tests, but had not. I met a woman who should have had screening tests for cardiac risk, and received select immunizations—who had not. I met a woman who had been driven from any and all benefits that modern medicine might offer her by the cold and denigrating judgment offered her by almost every modern medical practitioner she had met.[15]

Putting all of this together, it seems that while there may not be any overt intention on the part of most physicians to discriminate against or to demean overweight and obese patients, the patients are able either to sense their physicians' underlying disapproval or project it upon them and cope with this by minimizing their interactions with physicians. Some of this implicit bias may have its source in the inclination of many to blame the patient for his disease whenever deviant or immoral behaviors are believed to be its cause, as was described earlier in chapter 4. While it is perhaps unsurprising that many healthcare professionals harbor the same inherent responses to conditions that they see as having been preventable, the fact that they do militates for a greater self-awareness about their possible presence and the need for conscious efforts to be made so as to overcome those biased responses.

HEALTH ILLITERACY AS A BARRIER TO PHYSICIAN-PATIENT COMMUNICATION

Another major impediment to physician-patient communication that often goes unidentified by physicians is *heath illiteracy*. Health literacy, defined by Ruth Parker, of Emory University, as "basic skills in reading, writing and numeracy . . . in the health care setting, where patient participation in planning and implementing therapeutic regimens is critical for success," encompasses a broad range of skills. She further explains: "Patients need to be able to understand oral and written information about their medical conditions, follow written and numerical directions regarding their therapeutic regimens and diagnostic tests, ask pertinent questions of medical personnel, report prior conditions and treatment, and solve problems that arise during the course of their care."[16]

Health illiteracy is more common a problem than perhaps most people, physicians included, realize. One study, which looked at the health literacy of Medicare patients enrolled in a large managed-care organization, found that almost 36 percent possessed "marginal" or "insufficient" health literacy skills. Low levels of health literacy are a risk factor for hospital readmissions shortly after discharge, poor medical adherence, and increased overall health-care costs. However, despite its widespread prevalence, many physicians do not look for it, and therefore do not recognize it, in their patients.[17]

Because of its high prevalence, a group of researchers introduced health-literacy screening with a tool called The Newest Vital Sign as part of the routine intake process in a family-medicine clinic serving a panel of more than 5,500 patients. The screening was done prior to the actual visit with the physician. The total startup and implementation costs were $11,800 during the year it was studied, and it demanded less than thirty seconds of each patient's time and less than two minutes on average for the administrative staff to enter each patient's results into the electronic health record. Physicians reported spending more time with those patients identified as having low health literacy, tailoring their instructions and directives to the patients' needs and confirming comprehension. Two-thirds of the physicians in that clinic reported that using this tool improved the quality of the care they provided to their patients.[18]

It's really important to stop and consider this from a systems perspective. Low health literacy is associated with additional health costs that have been calculated to be as high as $7,800 *per patient per year.*[19] The implementation and management coasts of health literacy screening for a busy clinic responsible for 5,500 patients were miniscule compared to that. Although the researchers did not assess outcomes measures as part of their study, it is highly likely that the savings to the health-care system as a whole were many times that of the initial investment, certainly with a patient panel of this size. This is because of the connection between improved patient understanding of treatment direction and goals, increased adherence, better outcomes, and reduced costs. Yet it is important to note that while the costs of implementation were borne by the medical practice itself in the form of uncompensated administrative and physician time, the actual savings that accrued from it went elsewhere. Without correcting this, even the relatively low implementation costs of an intervention such as this will serve as a powerful disincentive to widespread adoption so long as they are not compensated for.

The problem of poor health literacy extends into the realm of medical decision making by patients as well, namely, being able to choose among different treatment options based upon an adequate understanding of their consequences. This is known as *informed consent*. Physicians are required to obtain informed consent before performing most medical procedures as well as certain treatments. Informed consent is important for ethical and legal reasons. Our society places a very high value on personal autonomy, and the requirement of informed consent is designed to protect patients against medical procedures or treatments that they might otherwise choose not to undergo because their true nature is misrepresented or because they are coerced into agreeing to them. Yet even when informed consent is given, it is to all practical purposes meaningless if the physician is unable to translate the potential risks and benefits into terms comprehensible to the patient. The physician, feeling at home in his specialty of biomedicine, may use professional jargon too liberally or simply provide more information than the patient can easily absorb. This is clearly obvious with complex medical procedures. However, it is also true for basic complications recognizable by name yet elusive in meaning until experienced because their very nature is so dissimilar to anything the patient has experienced before. Take pain, for example. Describing the aftereffects of the radiation therapy he underwent to treat his esophageal cancer, Christopher Hitchens wrote:

Every time I did swallow, a hellish tide of pain would flow up my throat, culminating in what felt like a mule kick in the small of my back. . . . [Pain is] impossible to warn against. If my proton physicians had tried to tell me up front, they might perhaps have spoken of "grave discomfort" or perhaps of a burning sensation. I only know that nothing at all could have readied or steadied me for this thing that seemed to scorn painkillers and to attack me in my core.[20]

Other factors that compromise the physician's ability truly to inform the patient can include the presence of language barriers, general illiteracy, and insufficient mental faculties on the part of the patient necessary to comprehend what is being said: for example, if the patient is developmentally delayed, mentally impaired, or suffering from dementia. Likewise, conditions of extreme stress can prove overwhelming for a patient, exceeding his capacity to make an informed decision. Describing his experience performing emergency caesarean sections in the middle of the night to Pam Belluck, author of *Island Practice*, Dr. Tim Lepore states emphatically: "you cannot obtain informed consent on a patient who is non-English speaking, has been medicated, and it's 3 o'clock in the morning. You tell me that that's informed consent, I'll say to you that that's bullshit."[21]

In an essay published in the *Journal of the American Medical Association*, the Boston University surgeon Eugene Laforet went so far as to suggest that the whole concept of informed consent was a fraud. "In the final analysis, regardless of whether society or the medical profession or the law wants it that way, the best, and probably only, guarantee of a patient's rights is the integrity of his physician," he wrote. Because it is impossible to obtain truly "informed" consent from a large segment of patients for reasons described above, Laforet concluded that in many cases "informed consent is a legalistic fiction that destroys good patient care and paralyzes the conscientious physician."[22]

I first became aware of how big the problem of health illiteracy was and how it related to patient medical decision making during the third year of my pediatric residency in Israel. I was about three hours into call at the neonatal intensive care unit (NICU) when my pager went off. Marina, the obstetrics resident covering the delivery room, was calling to let me know that she had a twenty-five-year-old woman who was twenty-seven weeks (six months) pregnant with twins, now in active labor, and who would probably deliver within the next hour.

"You'd better call your attending at home and tell her to come in," she said. "I'm sorry, Dennis. You're not going to get much sleep tonight."

She was right.

Forty minutes later my attending and I received the twins, immediately inserting straw-sized endotracheal tubes into their windpipes right there in the delivery suite, and spraying surfactant into their immature lungs to help them breathe. Once that was taken care of, we placed them inside the prewarmed incubators and rolled them back to the NICU for further care, each securing with our left hands one of the babies' endotracheal tubes so that it wouldn't become dislodged in transit, and squeezing breaths of oxygen-enriched air from specially sized AMBU bags into the babies' lungs with our right. After we transferred the babies to the open-air incubators in the NICU, we proceeded to thread long, thin catheters into their umbilical veins so that they could be given intravenous fluids, antibiotics, and medications. Other catheters went into their umbilical arteries so that we could monitor their blood pressure and draw blood for labs without having to stick them multiple times and increase their risk of infection. We adjusted the ventilators that controlled their breathing and made sure their body temperatures were stable and that their kidneys were producing enough urine. We fiddled with and repositioned their tubes and lines while simultaneously fielding questions from the nurses about the other ten babies in the unit, two of whom were "dynamic" that evening and required frequent changes made to their care.

It's easy to lose track of time when you're busy, and the sheer volume of data that kept coming my way about the tiny boy I was responsible for kept me occupied for close to ninety minutes. At a certain point, though, things seemed OK, and he seemed to have stabilized. Looking up from the open incubator and stretching my neck, I removed my gloves and turned around to face to my attending, who was still working on my baby's sister.

"Ada, do you need a hand?"

"No, thanks," she said without looking up. "I've got things under control." And then: "Perhaps you can go outside and update the family. They're probably wondering what's going on with these two."

Stepping through the accordion-like partition that served as the door between the NICU and the Newborn Unit, I saw about fifteen people. Half a dozen men were deep in conversation, their *tzitziyot* (ritually prescribed fringes) dangling down from under their white shirts and the black velvet *kippot* (yarmulkes) on their heads identifying them as orthodox Jews. One, in his mid-twenties, appeared to be the twins' father, judging from his bewildered expression, and next to him were two older men who, I later learned, were the twins' grandfathers. Off to the side, a man in his mid-forties was speaking softly into a cellphone as he leaned against the wall, his left shoulder partially obscuring the sign forbidding the use of cellphones near the NICU. On the other side sat a group of women engaged in animated conversation about their own birth experiences and about whether or not they'd be able to celebrate a *brit mila* for the boy in eight days. On the ceiling above, the long fluorescent lamp flickered erratically, out of synch with the sounds from the monitors that carried across the flimsy partition and that were the only indication (to those who knew how to interpret them) of the medical dramas taking place just a few steps away. There was the scent of curried rice that one of the nurses in the Newborn Unit had heated for her dinner, but it could not completely mask the underlying smell of amniotic fluid and childbirth, which was always the first thing I noticed whenever I came into the pavilion.

At first, the only person who seemed to notice me was the older man on the cellphone, who nodded at me as if to signal he'd be off the phone in just a moment and then turned away. Then the father saw me, identifying me as a physician, I'm sure, by the scrubs I was wearing.

He took one step toward me, then stopped. It was as if unsure he was unsure what to do or even to say.

"*Heenay hadoktor higi'a!* [The doctor has arrived!]," exclaimed one of the women, and then, all at once, three of them stood up and made their way toward me. The other women and the men followed, forming a half-circle around me. A woman who looked to be in her mid-forties wearing a dark kerchief on her head, a red cardigan, and long patterned skirt and who carried herself like the matriarch of the group (she was, in fact, the mother of the twins' mother) took center position. She asked me how the babies were.

It felt really good, standing there and telling them about all that my attending and I had done for the infants. I described how we had received the babies, intubated and ventilated them, and stabilized their breathing. I explained how we had given them medicines to keep their blood pressures steady. I reviewed with satisfaction the head ultrasounds we'd done, which did not show evidence of bleeding. I informed them that the girl had a heart murmur and that while we'd get an ECHO cardiogram to confirm, it was likely the result of a blood vessel that might close on its own, and that if it didn't, we might need to give her medicine to do that or even consider surgery. I felt so smart and important standing there and was really enjoying showing off my command of medicine to these people whose newest family members my attending and I had just saved. Yes, I was bragging and showing off. But it doesn't feel like bragging when it's true.

For at least ten seconds after I finished speaking, they all just stood there, staring at me silently with unreadable expressions on their faces. Even now, I'm not sure what I was expecting to hear from them. Fawning admiration? A grudging concession that science was more powerful than religion, that Fanaroff's neonatology textbook trumped the Talmud? Applause? Whatever it might have been, that wasn't what I got. I was completely taken aback by the grandmother's next question:

"*Aval doktor, kama hem shoklim?* [But doctor, how much do they weigh?]"

The longer I've been in practice and the more time I've spent with patients and their families, the more I understand not only about where that question came from but also what it says about much of the "dialogue of the deaf" that all too often passes for communication between physicians and patients. These people weren't stupid; nor were they by any means disengaged from the modern world which surrounded them. However, they were also in no position to make sense out of the myriad data and factoids I had just bombarded them with. The one measure of the newborns' well-being that they could relate to, the single most important piece of information that they needed in order to contextualize the infants' condition within their personal and collective experiences and that they could share with others, was exactly that which I had neglected to provide them with: the infants' birth weight. If the babies weighed less than four pounds—and in fact, they weighed less than two pounds each—the *brit mila* would need to be postponed. All the rest could have been science fiction as far as they were concerned.

The complexities of modern medicine, with its ion channels, magnetic resonance imaging, and proton knives are simply too abstract for most laypeople to comprehend (and this includes many physicians who do not encounter these things regularly in their own practices). And indeed, had I asked them at that moment to consent to an operation to correct the girl's heart defect, it is hard to see how they could have provided anything remotely "informed," other than by how I would have chosen to present the clinical scenario and options for treatment and that would have reflected my own inclinations and not their independent decision.

I'd like to conclude this chapter with a passage written by Irwin Press in 1981, at the time a professor of anthropology at Notre Dame University:

The ideal biomedical health practitioner should be expert in theology, anthropology, psychology and urban studies. This is another way of noting that societal, cultural, ideological and contextual phenomena necessarily express themselves in all aspects of human behavior, and that episodes of disease are not excepted. Of course, no physician, nurse, or other biomedical practitioner can meet these requirements. However, it can be argued that the more aware such practitioners are of the operation of cultural factors in the expression and cure of disease, the more capable they will be of dealing with their culture-bearing patients.[23]

I couldn't agree more. In a perfect world, physicians would be omnipotent and blessed with insight and understanding in all of these fields (and more!), enabling them to communicate better with their patients and with deeper empathy and understanding. In the real world, however, where we all have our own individual strengths and weaknesses and are under pressure from all directions, it takes more than just wishing for good things to make them happen. Actions, too, are necessary, as I'll describe in the final two chapters.

7

MAKING IT STICK

'Tis not enough to help the feeble up, but to support him after.

—William Shakespeare, *Timon of Athens*

IN THE previous chapters of this book, I've shown how differences in cultural frameworks and belief systems can result in significant miscommunication between patients and their physicians. However, even when both speak the same language—literally and metaphorically—the presence of such factors as pain, fear, and emotional stress, which accompany almost every patient-physician interaction to one degree or another, can lead to significant misunderstanding, on the part of the patient, of what she is being told by her physician. The resulting confusion can be especially momentous when it extends to treatment recommendations and have far-reaching consequences for the patient's health and well-being.

THE POWER OF THE WRITTEN WORD

As I mentioned earlier in chapter 1, several years ago I herniated two discs in my lower back. The injury caused me severe and prolonged pain and kept me from standing fully upright and from lying down flat for almost three months. My primary-care physician referred me to an orthopedic back specialist who examined both me and my MRI. As in so many other cases, the MRI had absolutely no bearing on my treatment, though I must say that on a personal level it did boost my morale considerably by providing objective "validity" to my suffering, which made me feel like much less of a wimp.

After she had assured me that there was no need for anything more than conservative management of my back injury, the back specialist prescribed me three different medications to control the inflammation, muscle spasm, and pain. I was familiar with all three even though I do not routinely prescribe them myself, and certainly never to treat this kind of injury. Still, I had a good general sense of what the appropriate doses were for each, how frequently they needed to be taken, whether or not they should be taken before or after meals, and what their potential side effects were. Or so I thought.

I listened carefully to what the back specialist told me, nodding my head in understanding . . . and found myself returning to her office only a few minutes after leaving, hopelessly confused. Embarrassed, I asked her physician assistant to review for me once again the precise instructions about how often the different meds were meant to be taken, and this time, I made sure to write everything out so that I could keep the instructions straight in my head. And it was a very good thing that I did!

Everything the back specialist had told me had gotten completely jumbled in my mind, probably because of the combination of pain and anxiety, which made it difficult for me to follow her instructions. Yet I'm sure that she had felt that I had understood everything she had said, even though I hadn't.

It was just like the scene from the movie *Monty Python and the Holy Grail* where the King of Swamp Castle locks his son in the tower and gives orders to the two guards standing watch outside:

KING OF SWAMP CASTLE: Guards, make sure the prince doesn't leave this room until I come and get him.
GUARD #1: Not to leave the room . . . even if you come and get him.
KING OF SWAMP CASTLE: No, no. *Until* I come and get him.
GUARD #1: Until you come and get him, we're not to enter the room.
KING OF SWAMP CASTLE: No, no. You *stay* in the room, and make sure *he* doesn't leave.

GUARD #1: And you'll come and get him.

KING OF SWAMP CASTLE: Right.

GUARD #1: We don't need to do anything, apart from just stop him entering the room.

KING OF SWAMP CASTLE: No, no, leaving the room.

GUARD #1: Leaving the room, yes.[1]

Even after I had left the back specialist's office for the second time, with my newly clarified instructions about how I was supposed to take the different medications I had just been prescribed, I remained concerned that I might become addicted to the narcotic painkillers, just as I had seen happen to patients I had cared for in the past. Most had become addicted to their meds because of poor guidance from their physicians about how to take them and not because of drug-seeking behavior. In retrospect I know that I could, and probably should, have used my own pain meds more liberally than I did to control better the often excruciating discomfort that plagued me for more than three months. But I was terrified by the possibility of becoming addicted, not least because of the vague instructions I had been given: *take one to two pills every six to eight hours as needed.* End of story. More precise guidance, including about how to avoid becoming dependent upon these medications, would have enabled me to make better use of them and afforded me greater relief from my pain.

According to the Centers for Disease Control and Prevention (CDC), there are 1.2 million emergency room visits each year because of the misuse and/or abuse of medications. The direct health-care costs of this have been calculated to be in excess of $72 billion *annually*. The medications most often misused are those whose very nature sets them up for it: narcotic pain relievers. In 2010, more than 22,000 Americans died because of prescription drug overdose, and slightly more than 75 percent of these deaths involved prescription-only narcotic pain-relief medication. The nonmedical abuse of narcotic pain relievers is very widespread—in 2010, almost 5 percent of Americans age twelve and older reported doing so—and very costly to society. While often obtained and used illicitly, in many cases these drugs are prescribed by well-intentioned physicians to treat their patients' complaints of chronic pain. All too often, however, patients are not given sufficiently clear guidance about how the meds should be taken and are not monitored closely enough for signs of developing addiction.[2]

My own experience with the back specialist helped me understand how completely wrongheaded I had been when I had grumbled about the requirement to provide written asthma-action plans (an instruction sheet detailing how and when the different medications prescribed to control a patient's asthma should be given, based upon the severity of symptoms) to my asthmatic patients at least once a year, as well as with every medication change. I could now see that asthma-action plans do indeed make a great deal of sense. If I, a physician, had become so confused about how I was meant to take three medications I was reasonably familiar with, how could I possibly expect my patients to fare any better, especially as the instructions for the medications I prescribe change in accordance with how sick the patient is? As I explored this more, I learned that providing written or printed instructions that reinforce what is discussed at our visits and that can be referred to for guidance if and when symptoms appear or worsen does indeed improve health outcomes for patients with asthma,[3] as well as for patients with any number of other conditions.

PROVIDING HANDOUTS AND DISCHARGE INSTRUCTIONS

We physicians can sometimes forget just how stressful it is for people to have to come and see us. After all, caring for unhealthy people and treating disease are what we do; it is a normal part of our lives. Most people, however, are *not* accustomed to being unhealthy, and if and when this happens to them they typically become worried and anxious, for good reason. This makes it very difficult for them to remember to ask their physicians all of the important questions they'd planned to and to process and remember the answers they receive. And even when the patient begins his visit with the physician in a relatively calm state, he can easily be thrown off balance by something the physician says or does, which is then seized upon and attributed special significance to, far beyond that intended by the physician. This then distracts the patient from whatever else is going on at the moment and interferes with his ability to absorb any further information.

I once cared for an adult patient who had developed mild kidney dysfunction during his hospitalization because of the antibiotics he was being given. One morning, when I went in to see him, I found him visibly agitated. When I asked what the matter was, he told me that the consulting nephrologist had just been by to see him and that he (the patient) had concluded that his condition was much graver than any of us, the nephrologist included, had been letting on. I hastened to reassure him that this was not the case and indeed was quite surprised to hear this, not least because I myself had spoken with the nephrologist only a few minutes earlier, and we had both agreed that my patient was making good progress. I then asked my patient what had led him to understand this about his condition. It turned out that the nephrologist's facial expressions, along with his use of the words "renal failure," had scared my patient into thinking that he was in imminent need of a kidney transplant, even though his kidney function was actually improving nicely. Now, it is true that that particular nephrologist—one of the most compassionate and dedicated people I know—doesn't smile often and tends to wear a rather concerned-looking facial expression. But I was amazed at how this, and the use of a technical term—renal failure—which sounded a lot worse than actually intended, had caused my patient to misunderstand fundamentally the nephrologist's assessment. It underscored for me once again the centrality of nonverbal communication between physician and patient and demonstrated how easily it can outweigh the actual content of the conversation.

Because stress, distraction, and lack of concentration caused by pain or medications can be present at any clinical interaction, it is very important to provide patients with information that they can return to after the clinical encounter for guidance and for reinforcement of what was discussed, both for acute and chronic disease. This can be provided in a variety of formats and media and improves both medical outcomes and patient satisfaction.[4]

Women at risk for premature delivery, for example, report better understanding of the long-term health risks of premature delivery to their children, as well as less overall anxiety, when provided with written handouts summarizing the prenatal counseling they've received. This is not surprising: most women in this situation are under tremendous stress and have never heard of many of the potential health problems being presented to them before, to say nothing of ever having had to deal with them before. In other situations, such as that of patients starting to resume daily activities following cataract surgery, illustrated instructions have been shown to be very effective in getting them to follow their physicians' recommendations. Pictographs have also been used effectively in the outpatient clinic setting to improve medication and dietary adherence in diabetic patients with low health literacy significantly. Likewise, mobile videos have been shown to be very useful in teaching patients how to carry out specific tasks, such as wound care, following discharge from the emergency room.[5]

CONFIRMING UNDERSTANDING

One setting in which it is especially commonplace for patients not to understand the instructions given to them by their physicians is the emergency room. Often times, they have just been diagnosed with a new condition that can involve hitherto unfamiliar treatments and that requires them to be attentive to details they had never really noticed before. Consider, for example, a fifty-year-old woman diagnosed with acute bronchitis in the emergency room and deemed healthy enough not to need hospitalization. She might be put on a ten-day course of twice-daily antibiotics and an inhaler, to be used four times a day; told to take ibuprofen for fever up to every six hours as needed; to watch her fluid intake; and to seek urgent medical care in the event of high fever, chest pain, or worsening shortness of breath. That's a lot to take in, especially when you're not feeling well.

As many as one out of every five return visits to the emergency room is the direct outcome of poor patient education. The two areas in which patients discharged from the emergency room report the most confusion are how to care for themselves at home and under which circumstances they need to return to the emergency room for further care. Because of this, discharge instructions are now provided by many emergency rooms as a matter of course.[6] However, they only solve part of the problem.

Researchers analyzing more than eight hundred discharges from two large emergency departments were amazed to find that in over three-quarters of the discharges, the medical team never confirmed that the patients had actually *understood* what they had been told. Likewise, a study done at the University of Michigan Department of Emergency Medicine found that although more than a quarter of the adults discharged from the ER did not comprehend significant portions of their discharge instructions, only 20 percent were even aware of this.[7] This meant that they didn't even know what questions to ask. As with so many other things in life, it is very hard to fix something you don't know is even broken.

When medical instructions are unsuited to a patient's learning style or to his or her general and/or health literacy levels, they alone will not be enough to improve health outcomes, such as, for example, reduced hospital readmissions. A recent review of thirty different asthma-action plans endorsed at the state or federal levels found that their overall readability exceeded a seventh-grade level, despite recommendations that patient-education materials not exceed a sixth-grade level.[8] This is why confirming that patients *understand* the medical instructions they are given is essential to them being carried out and, ultimately, to achieving the desired outcomes.

One of the best ways of verifying comprehension is through the *teach-back* method, in which the physician asks her patient to repeat the instructions back to her. Not only does this allow the physician to make sure that the instructions were understood, but it also provides the patient with an opportunity to ask questions and request clarifications. This can help identify patients who may have difficulties with language proficiency or health literacy and who require extra assistance such as interpreter services, teaching aids in a simpler language, or ones that rely more on graphic images.[9]

There is often a temptation to skip over teach-backs, especially when the clinic (or emergency room, or hospital ward) is busy and the physician does not immediately sense that her patient has difficulty understanding her instructions. However, this impression can often be false, as it is very easy to conflate general literacy skills with health literacy. Likewise, as I noted in the previous chapter, physicians can find it quite challenging to accurately identify health-illiterate patients in the absence of targeted screening.[10]

As someone who prescribes asthma medications on almost a daily basis, for example, nothing could seem more intuitive to me than using these meds correctly. Yet, as I need to remind myself regularly, it is precisely *because* I prescribe them so frequently that knowing how to use them seems so straightforward to me. Even if my patients, their parents, and I are able to carry on in-depth conversations about non-medical interests we share, that provides no indication that when it comes to asthma management, they'll intuitively understand how and when to use medication A, at what frequency and at what dose, versus when to use medication B. This is perhaps the most delicate and important stage of the visit, so this is where I need to be the most vigilant and to take full responsibility that everything I say is understood by my patients and their parents, no matter how intelligent or medically savvy they are. My own experience with the back specialist illustrates this perfectly.

A few years ago, researchers from UCLA analyzed 181 patient visits in which a total of 234 new medications were prescribed by family physicians, internists, and cardiologists in southern California. They found that the average time spent by the physicians educating their patients about each new medication was . . . forty-nine seconds![11] And yes, it really *is* very difficult to cover all of these aspects of the medical management of disease in just forty-nine seconds. Even the Swamp King from *Monty Python and the Holy Grail* spent ninety-six seconds explaining to his guards what he wanted, and they still didn't get it.

IMPROVING ADHERENCE

It's not enough that medications be taken as scheduled: they also need to be taken *correctly*. With my asthmatic patients who require inhaled medications to keep their symptoms under control, making sure that they're taking their medications with proper technique is a critical part of what I do. If they aren't, instead of going into the lungs, the aerosolized medications stick to the insides of the patient's mouth and wind up being swallowed, taken far away from the lungs and unable to do what they are supposed to. Not only does this mean that the metered-dose inhalers (puffers) need to be used with spacers,[12] but it also means that the patients need to stand while inhaling, take an appropriate number of breaths with each puff, hold their breath for a certain number of seconds, etc. I've learned that asking the parent (or child, if old enough) to walk me through every step of how the medicines are given and/or taken is a very important part of our visit together and that, in most cases, there are details that need tweaking. This is as true for patients whom I have been following for years as it is for new patients. Often, a patient's internal family dynamic has changed (a new sibling has been born, a parent who had been at home has now returned to work), or more of the responsibility for taking the medications has shifted to the child himself as he grows older. Because of this, the parent may simply be unaware that they are either no longer being taken as they should be or why they are not.[13]

For example, many parents of children with asthma whose symptoms are triggered by exercise believe that their children take their inhaled medication before gym class just as we've discussed, without actually verifying that this is indeed so. When they see their child unable to play more than ten minutes of basketball without becoming short of breath, they assume that this means that their child is sicker, that the medicines are no longer working, and that their child needs to be on something stronger. Often, however, it turns out that the real problem is that their kid is embarrassed to use her inhaler with the spacer in front of her friends because she thinks it makes her look "dorky." Finding a way to help her slip off unnoticed to the school nurse's office ten minutes before gym class so that she can take her medicine unobserved is a lot more effective than yelling at her that she needs to take her medicine *or else*. It is also certainly better than switching her to a different medication with an unnecessarily higher side-effect profile.

Although it is beyond the scope of this book, it is important to mention that using certain communication styles within the physician-patient interview can make a big difference in patient adherence with treatment regimens. One of these is known as "motivational interviewing." This is a communication strategy that departs from a physician-patient dynamic characterized by interrogation followed by (mostly unidirectional) information transmission from the physician to the patient. Motivational interviewing is more nuanced and relies much more upon the physician asking open-ended questions and reflecting the answers back to the patient. As Rollnick, Miller, and Butler write in their book *Motivational Interviewing in Health Care*, it is much easier to enlist the collaboration of a patient to change his illness behaviors in response to internal motivation rather than to external pressure. Once the patient "owns" the decision to make the prescribed change (weight loss, quitting smoking, etc.), he is much more likely to follow through than if he feels he needs to so because "that's what the doctor ordered." They advocate identifying the patient's desires, needs, abilities, and reasons for making the changes in illness behavior that are necessary for better adherence and overall health and turning these into the prime motivators which prompt the patient to do so. The technique of motivational interviewing improves adherence in patients being treated for substance abuse, diabetes, and weight loss, among other conditions, and also effectively helps to reduce HIV-risk behavior.[14]

SHARED MEDICAL DECISION MAKING

Just as identifying and drawing upon a patient's primary motivators increases adherence, so too does tailoring a patient's treatments to her specific needs and characteristics—through a process of shared medical decision making—make it more likely that they will be carried out successfully.[15] Doing so entails bidirectional communication and negotiation between physician and patient, without the physician ceding her authority, which is based upon her medical knowledge and experience. The very process of sharing medical decisions provides the physician with valuable insights into potential obstacles to medical adherence that could easily be avoided without compromising the efficacy of the treatments.

Earlier, in chapter 2, I discussed shared medical decision making in the context of end-of-life care. However, that is only one small area in which shared medical decision making effectively improves health outcomes and reduces medical costs. This isn't just because of improved adherence, though that, too, is important. It turns out that most patients are fully capable of making rational, well-thought-out decisions that affect their own health when they are presented with and able to understand the information upon which to base them.

Active patient participation in the medical decision-making process is possible only when the patient understands the choices and their implications. In some instances, these are relatively straightforward and easy to comprehend: whether or not to amputate the gangrenous foot of a diabetic patient, for example. Others are much more nuanced, such as whether or not to aggressively treat early-stage prostate cancer. While many patients, especially older ones, may prefer to leave the medical decision making squarely in the hands of their physicians, they may still be able to provide a lot of information to the physician about their preferences, even when these are expressed deferentially or indirectly.[16]

One way of looking at medical decision making is by distinguishing a predominantly analytical decision-making process based primarily upon data from one in which emotions, heuristics, and values play equally important roles. This is known as naturalistic, or "whole-mind," decision making. When physician and patient share in this process of whole-mind decision making, it is referred to as "shared-mind" decision making. In this schema, the role of the physician is not only to provide data to the patient for analytical consideration but also to help the patient identify how his quality of life will be directly affected by the different therapeutic options he must choose from, even in ways he may be completely unaware of. When the physician helps the patient do so, the patient is then able to utilize a whole-mind decision-making process to make the best choices about his own care.[17] The story of my interaction with Isabelle and her family, which I shared in chapter 2, is an example of whole-mind/shared-mind decision making, in which the decision about whether or not to proceed with a trache was much more than merely a medical one and required the integration of the family's values and overall goals of care.

With the majority of patients desiring to be more involved in the decisions about their own care, such as which medications they should be on, for example, the default should be to do so.[18] This doesn't mean that patients who ask for antibiotics when they are inappropriate should be prescribed them with abandon, but it appears that in many instances, adopting a model of shared medical decision making between physicians and patients renders that point moot. A recent Canadian study found that the patients of family physicians who had undergone training in shared medical decision making were almost 50 percent less likely to use antibiotics for respiratory tract infections than the patients of physicians who hadn't undergone the training.[19] Again, it was the *physicians* who had received the training, not the patients, yet there was clearly something about the physicians' style of interaction with their patients and the heightened sense of implicit trust it bred that resulted in a better and more judicious use of antibiotics.

In order to promote shared medical decision making, decision aids are increasingly being introduced into clinical practice. A recent study published in *Health Affairs* looked at the effects of health coaching via different media aimed at encouraging patients to become more actively involved in making their own medical decisions. The researchers found that this resulted in a greater than 5 percent savings in cost, a greater than 12 percent reduction in hospitalizations, and in almost 10 percent fewer preference-driven surgical procedures. In pediatrics, shared medical decision making between the parents of children with special needs and their physicians has been shown to significantly reduce emergency room visits, hospitalizations, and overall medical costs for these kids. Another study found that the use of medical decision-making aids by orthopedic patients who were members of a large health-care system in the northwestern United States led to a 26 and 38 percent reduction, respectively, in hip- and in knee-replacement surgeries. To put this in perspective, in 2010 alone, there were more than 650,000 hip replacements and 250,000 knee replacements done in the United States, at an annual cost of $15.6 billion.[20]

Although physicians are required to promote shared medical decision making in order to participate in Medicare's Shared Savings Program, many resist doing so. One study examining the use of decision-making aids in everyday practice found that these were only being used in 10 to 30 percent of the opportunities they could have been. One of the barriers identified by many physicians was the perception that using them takes up too much time.[21] However, this most certainly need not be the case, as medical decision-making aids can be deployed at any time during the medical encounter and do not need to be restricted to the actual time spent with the physician. This is something that I'll discuss in greater detail in chapter 8. Utilized prior to the visit with the physician, medical decision-making aids can not only help the patient consider the pros and cons of various options but also help the patient formulate questions that can then be answered by the physician during the visit itself. Used after the visit, either while the patient is still in the clinic or at home, they can serve as a source of information that can be repeatedly referenced while the patient deliberates about what choice would be best for him.

THE IMPORTANCE OF PHYSICIAN-PATIENT FACE TIME

The value of physician time must be considered in any serious discussion of how to contain the inexorable rise of health-care expenditures in this country. As I'm sure is obvious, I believe that in order for physicians to perform their healing task to the best of their abilities, they must be able to devote to their patients the time necessary to do so adequately. Unfortunately, this premise is increasingly being challenged in the name of so-called efficiency. With that said, it is also true that many of the tasks currently performed by physicians could easily be done by others. These include the routine intake of information, patient education, prescription management, and adherence monitoring. Doing this would involve the transfer of certain components of routine medical care to other health-care professionals within the same care-provision framework, with physicians assuming more of a supervisory role for these tasks. This would free up more time for physicians to spend on those tasks that only they are qualified to do. They would be able to spend more time with their patients and perhaps expand the total number of patients they see. This is a different approach toward making physicians and health-care provision in general more efficient, and it will be discussed in greater detail in chapter 8.

The offloading of some of the traditional responsibilities of physicians onto other health-care providers is already starting to take place in the outpatient setting, especially in primary care, where physician assistants and nurse practitioners play an expanding role in direct patient care. The same is true in operating rooms across the country, where certified registered nurse anesthetists provide thirty-two million anesthetics annually.[22] Further expanding the scope of practice of so-called physician extenders within the health-care system so that the challenges of caring for an aging and more medically complex population can be met will require changing how efficiency in health care is defined and compensated for. In contrast to the logic of the fee-for-service paradigm, in which efficiency is measured by the number of patients seen or procedures done within a certain time frame, efficiency would need to be redefined as value produced per unit of spending or time, in this case that of the physician. This would entail designating value as a function of health outcomes divided by cost, assessing these outcomes with metrics based primarily upon measures of *health*, not throughput (number of patients seen per hour of physician time), and by reducing the overall utilization of medical services without compromising health-outcome measures. This appears to be the direction we are headed in with the movement toward the assumption of global risk by vertically oriented accountable-care organizations, in which payment is disbursed to providers by third-party payors on a global per-patient basis, stratified by complexity, irrespective of the individual services actually consumed. However, there is a fine line between reducing the unnecessary utilization of health-care services and cutting back on the time—and services—that are needed to get the job actually done right. Although most physicians and patients recognize this, there are others who, dazzled by the short-term gain that having physicians see more patients in the same amount of time can yield, seem oblivious to the associated costs—direct and indirect—that will necessarily arise from the more hurried and less effective communication between physician and patient.

This point is vitally important, and affects all of us.

Although it might sound revolutionary within the American health-care system circa 2014, it's worth considering how sensible it is in virtually every other industry. You certainly wouldn't think that your auto mechanic was better simply because he could get the job done in one hour instead of three, if it also meant that you had to take the car back to the garage two more times that week before you could actually drive it safely. Why should it be any different in health care? If your physician is able to take the extra time to make the correct diagnosis by taking a careful history and doing a thorough physical examination, you'd doubtlessly prefer that to being in and out in twenty minutes and sent off for a battery of tests, many unnecessary, uncomfortable, and expensive. And as I've already pointed out, physicians who spend more time with their patients *do* wind up ordering fewer tests and delivering less expensive care.[23]

Unfortunately, however, physicians are under increasing pressure to see more patients in less time, with predictable results. It begins for many during their training, with duty-hour restrictions that limit the number of hours they can be on the wards. Because this necessarily reduces the amount of time that work can be squeezed into, rather than the workload itself, compromises are made that often affect physician-patient communication. A recent study of two different internal-medicine training programs found that the interns spent just 12 percent of their time engaging with patients and directly involved in their care. In comparison, the interns spent more than *three times* that much time at computer work stations.[24]

The medical complexity of their patients, attributable, in part, to the ability of modern medicine to keep sicker people alive for longer, leaves many physicians with less time to address their patients' needs. One analysis of 392 primary-care physician visits found that a median number of *six* separate topics were covered during visits that spanned a median of 15.7 minutes. The main topic in each visit received about five minutes of attention; the other five received a little over a minute each.[25] That's an impossibly short amount of time to address thoroughly anything at all.

To provide better practical guidance to their patients, some physicians are beginning to adopt a model of shared medical appointments for patients with common diagnoses such as diabetes, for example.

These meetings, lasting for two hours, are led by a physician and a nurse and may include as many as twelve patients who share the same diagnosis. The visits may include a full physical examination of each patient done in private, or a simultaneous, targeted examination of one specific body part of everyone participating. This might consist of asking everyone to remove their shoes and socks so that their feet can be examined, allowing for communal discussion of foot care, a common concern in diabetic patients. The participants all sign confidentiality agreements, and although many patients report initial discomfort with the idea, the increasing popularity of this model testifies to its success.[26] The discussions at these meetings, which pertain to the common diagnosis shared by all the participants, allow for the transmission of the same relevant information to all of them at once, avoiding the need for repetition a dozen times over. The questions posed by the participants have the added value of approaching the same issue from many angles, which in itself can help overcome differences in understanding stemming from differences in culture, explanatory models of disease, and illness behavior. These questions, and the answers to them, also provide patients with an opportunity to hear about aspects of their disease and its management that might never have occurred to them otherwise.

One other field in which time constraints drive care in directions that do not always suit the best interests of patients is psychiatry, a discipline that has become much more medication oriented in recent years, mainly because falling reimbursement rates have made talk therapy poorly remunerative. It is unclear whether medications produce better outcomes than talk therapy in the treatment of many psychiatric disorders, such as depression, for example, which are now routinely medicated. This is very concerning, as the side-effect profiles of many of these medications are one of the main reasons for poor adherence, with relapse as well as suicide being major concerns in these patients.[27]

External interference in the structure and content of physician visits with patients and an increasingly oppressive administrative workload also serve to curtail the time necessary for good communication between physicians and patients to thrive. One reason that physicians have so little time to focus on patient concerns and problems is that they are increasingly obligated to attend to things wholly unrelated to the health issues that bring the patient in to see them in the first place. For example, physicians whose notes do not clearly state that they have performed a full review of systems may have their payment claims downgraded or denied altogether by third-party payors. The time a physician has for each visit is finite, which means that time used for one purpose necessarily comes at the expense of another. Consider, for example, a patient who comes in because she needs counseling on how to be more successful at using a new medical device she was recently prescribed. Teaching her how to use it properly is often what will determine whether or not she will ultimately succeed, be adherent with it, and benefit from it as a result. On the face of it, there is no reason why her physician should have to divert precious time away from doing so to ask whether she's noticed any recent changes in her vision, not because it has any particular relevance to her care but simply so that he can justify being paid for his time.

Dealing with the bureaucratic aspects of the practice of medicine such as billing and insurance devours a large amount of physician time and cuts into that time available for them to spend with their patients. A recent analysis of a large multistate medical group found that *each clinician* required a two-thirds of a full-time administrative staffperson's time to manage their billing and insurance paperwork. Even with this support, clinicians still spent over thirty-five minutes per day—almost three hours each week—dealing with bureaucratic matters. The annual cost per full-time clinician has been calculated as exceeding $85,000.[28] Simplifying this would not only reduce cost; it would also enable physicians to see more patients.

Physicians also spend a lot of time on patient care beyond the confines of the actual patient visits. One study looking at the between-visit workload of primary-care physicians in the Department of Veterans Affairs' health system found that this amounted to almost eight hours per week beyond the thirty-six hours of face time they were spending with patients. Eighty-two percent of this additional time—for which the physicians were not compensated—was spent managing patient care.[29] It is important to recognize this, as the pressure in many circles bearing down on physicians to see more patients uses as its calculus physician-patient face time and not the overall time required for patient care. This additional 22 percent of extraclinical time that needs to be spent on patient care beyond the actual visit—and in addition to the administrative time discussed above—cannot simply be ignored. Unless this time is accounted and budgeted for, something else will necessarily have to give: research, education, and the quality of patient care.

THE DOUBLE-EDGED SWORD OF HEALTH-INFORMATION TECHNOLOGY (HIT)

In 2000 the Institute of Medicine (IOM) released its now-famous report *To Err Is Human*, shocking Americans with its estimate that between 44,000 and 98,000 people die annually because of preventable medical errors.[30] To put those numbers into perspective, the authors wrote in their executive summary that "more people die in a given year as a result of medical errors than from motor vehicle accidents (43,458), breast cancer (42,297), or AIDS (16,516)." They also noted:

> Two out of every one-hundred admissions [to the hospital] experienced a preventable adverse drug event (ADE), resulting in average increased hospital costs of $4,700 per admission or about $2.8 million annually for a 700-bed teaching hospital. If these findings are generalizable, the increased hospital costs alone of preventable adverse drug events affecting inpatients are about $2 billion for the nation as a whole.[31]

A follow-up report by the IOM, issued in 2006, revised upward by 75 percent to $3.5 billion the previous estimate of the annual cost of adverse drug events in the hospital setting.[32] This, of course, is only a fraction of the cost to society, as most health care is provided in the outpatient setting.

Good communication between physicians and patients plays an important role in reducing the incidence of adverse events within the hospital setting, such as wrong-side surgery and medication errors. In most cases, these errors are caused not by negligence or carelessness but are almost the inevitable product of structural flaws within a system almost designed to fail. Following the release of *To Err Is Human* and its revelations about the unacceptable scale of medical error in the United States, many advocated integrating health-information technology (HIT) into medical practice to reduce both error and cost. A report issued by the RAND Corporation in 2005 estimated that if most hospitals and physicians' offices adopted HIT, the savings generated would exceed $77 billion per year.[33]

HIT is an umbrella term describing the medical use of information technology; it does not refer to a specific system or interface. The potential benefits of HIT in medicine are manifold. HIT allows for retrieval of vital information in real time about the patient's past medical history, medication utilization, immunization records, and allergies. The latter is especially important in situations where the physician caring for a particular patient has not met him before and/or the patient's ability to communicate is impaired. Both situations are commonly encountered in the emergency room, for example. HIT allows physicians more immediate access to lab results and imaging studies. HIT also can make medication prescription safer by printing prescriptions legibly and by identifying dosing errors, potential drug interactions, and allergies *before* the prescriptions are even filled.

In 2009, Congress passed the American Recovery and Reinvestment Act (ARRA), allocating up to $27 billion dollars to promote the adoption of electronic health records (EHR) and setting out financial incentives for physicians and hospitals adopting EHR and demonstrating "meaningful use."[34] These incentives range from tens of thousands of dollars to individual physicians to several million dollars each for hospitals. Along with the carrot of incentives came the stick of sanction: ARRA also stipulated reductions in reimbursements to physicians and hospitals not making the transition to EHR by 2015.

Even before ARRA was signed into law, the American health-care system had begun to adopt EHR. According to researchers from the Centers for Disease Control and Prevention's National Center for Health Statistics, just over 50 percent of nonfederal office-based physicians in the United States were using some form of EHR in 2010, up from 17.3 percent in 2002. Although encouraging, only 10.1 percent were using what was described as a "fully functional system," including features such as medication lists, physician notes, and patient problem lists; electronic prescription with real-time warnings about possible drug interactions and/or contraindications; warnings about abnormal lab test values; and guideline-based interventions or screening tests.[35]

While HIT has improved some health-outcomes, it is still unclear whether or not it actually has resulted in cost savings, especially those predicted by the RAND Corporation report. Indeed, there is evidence that HIT may actually be responsible for *increased* health-care costs. One study, which reviewed the outcomes of 28,741 patient visits with 1,187 physicians, found that physicians were 40 to 70 percent more likely to order additional imaging studies and 50 percent more likely to order additional blood tests when they had computerized access to the results of the original studies. Between the time the RAND report was issued in 2005 and the end of 2012, the annual expenditure on health care in the United States increased by $800 billion, or 40 percent. Whether or not this would have been higher or lower without HIT is unknown.[36]

Increasingly rigorous administrative oversight by third-party payors requires extensive documentation to satisfy them that services billed for by physicians were indeed provided to patients. Much of this documentation consists of standardized language that often hides important and clinically relevant information.[37] Not only does this not translate into better care for the patient; it wastes valuable time that physicians would otherwise use for actually seeing and caring for patients. To save time, many physicians resort to charting their visits during the appointments. This leads many physicians to spend a large portion of their visit time performing data entry and recovery, their eyes glued to the computer screen instead of regarding their patients. This in turn severely limits their ability to identify and respond to their patients' nonverbal cues and communication and to provide their own in response. Anne Marie Valinoti, an internist from New Jersey, recently wrote in the *Wall Street Journal* that using the EHR "may be getting in the way of meaningful encounters with our patients. With all the data entry the electronic system requires, my laptop presents a barrier between my patient and me, both physically and metaphorically. It's hard to be both stenographer and empathetic listener at the same time."[38]

Some researchers have found that physicians using an EHR are less likely to explore patient psychosocial and emotional issues and to discuss how the patients' lives are being affected by their health problems (i.e., illness) than those not using an EHR.[39] This discrepancy may be because of the more rigid structure imposed on the medical visit by the EHR, which, when used as a template for the visit itself, can interfere with the natural flow of the visit and especially the interview, breaking it down into discrete segments that follow a predetermined order. And although the sequence may be logical and applicable to most patients and to the narrative processes they employ to explain their complaints to the physician, it may be totally unsuited for others. This is especially true when the associations these patients draw between their symptoms and past medical history, diet, and so on are different than those the physician is accustomed to and/or when their cultural sensibilities make it difficult for patients to reveal what brought them to the physician in the first place. When this is the case, trying to fit a proverbial square peg into a round hole may lead to pieces breaking off, with important information not making it into the EHR.

Physicians and patients have, unsurprisingly, reported mixed reactions to the use of EHR in their visits. The positives reported by physicians include the immediacy with which test results and notes from other physicians within their network can be accessed and the time saved gathering information by no longer having to leaf through paper charts and inboxes or making phone calls and trips to the labs. Patients have reported satisfaction at improved communication among the various physicians caring for them. Communication about patients between the office staff and physicians through the EHR reduces interruptions to office flow. Physicians report being pleased at being able to provide easily accessible educational materials that can be tailored to fit their specific needs and those of their patients.[40]

However, physicians also note downsides to using an EHR. Chief among them is their own propensity to become distracted by the computer and the near-constant flow of new information coming through, most of it unrelated to the patient actually seated opposite them. This cuts to the heart of medical culture. Physicians are trained to intervene when something is not right, whether that something is an abnormal test result or an e-mailed summary of a visit that another patient had with a consultant that contains impressions and recommendations. Just as some check their phone every time it vibrates to announce a new e-mail, many physicians find it very tempting to click on their inbox each time their computer beeps to make sure that nothing important has come in that needs to be acted upon. This, of course, distracts tremendously from the patient in the room and the reasons that brought her to the clinic in the first place. One physician was quoted by the researchers as saying that using the EHR during patient visits is "like having a two-year-old in the room." Some patients complain that physicians who have computers in their clinic rooms spend less time in conversation and maintain less eye contact than before. Interestingly, patients also report that the physical examinations that were done were shorter and less comprehensive and that the visits felt less personal than those done in rooms without computers. Other patients have reported that the presence of computers in clinic rooms has either no effect or a positive one on their interactions with their physicians.[41] In this context it is important to note that while reconfiguring the clinic space can make it more likely that computers will facilitate, not hinder, communication between physician and patient, when computers do become a distraction, the problem is with how the physician uses them and not with the computers themselves.

The abundance of information available within the EHR has also led some physicians to say that they feel they spend less time actually conversing with their patients; others describe replacing open-ended questions in their interviews with standardized checklists. Some comment that there is a growing temptation to treat the patient's lab results instead of treating the patient. One physician told a researcher that "my concern now is that we're listening less because we have more information when we walk in the room, and it's not all trustworthy."[42]

OTHER USES OF HIT

The use of an EHR, however, is only one of many HIT innovations that are changing how physicians and patients communicate with one another. More and more, these interactions are occurring electronically. The pervasiveness of e-mail, smartphones, instant messaging, and social media has made communication between patients and physicians both easier and more difficult. Strict privacy regulations limit the information physicians are able to provide through these media, as do medicolegal and reimbursement considerations. Many patients resent these limitations, not understanding why it is that they must miss work and/or pull their kids out of school to go to the physician's office for something that could easily be resolved by e-mail. (This annoys many physicians as well.) For certain issues, the advantages of providing guidance by e-mail are clear, both from the physician-time and patient-time perspective. A Norwegian study that analyzed physician e-mail habits found that the mean time spent on each e-mail was a little more than two minutes.[43] While the minutes can quickly add up, e-mail communication will remain a much more convenient option for many patients, and making better use of it would free up physician time for patients with more serious issues who need to be seen in person. For this truly to succeed, however, the reimbursement and security aspects governing its use will need to be resolved. Also, it's important to remember that e-mail is an imperfect communication tool in many situations and that it can actually exacerbate miscommunication. Not only does e-mail not provide the visual cues present in face-to-face communication, but it lacks aural cues such as tone, emphasis, and prosody, as anyone who has ever been drawn into a spiral of misunderstood e-mails knows all too well.

The pitfalls of e-mail communication between physicians and patients were demonstrated by a study in which fifty physicians were asked to respond to an e-mail from a hypothetical patient. Although 92 percent of the physicians correctly identified the need to attend urgently to the patient's needs, based upon what was described in the e-mail, only 30 percent actively tried to get in touch with the patient.[44] This inattentiveness to the serious nature of the patient's e-mail may be because of how easy it is to access e-mail while on the go via smartphone (and then to forget about it the moment a new distraction comes along), or perhaps because the absence of visual and aural cues prevented the patient's message from crossing the physicians' inner threshold and triggering urgent action.

Telemedicine, the provision of medical care from afar facilitated by advanced monitoring and by audio and video technologies, has great potential for disseminating medical resources to geographically distant areas in which specialty care would otherwise be unavailable. However, it too has its limitations, not least of which is that actually meeting and choosing our physicians based upon our trust in their competence, manner, and values remain extremely important to us as patients. Although we may not mind having our EKG or chest X ray read by a physician sitting in an office in the next building or at a medical institution that we trust but that happens to be located in the next town over, we may not feel as comfortable when this is done from another country. Likewise, although treatment in intensive-care units provided remotely by physicians who monitor patients' status via computer and video feed may provide excellent outcomes,[45] never meeting, or being examined by, the physicians overseeing their care can be disconcerting and disturbing to many patients.

The farther away the physician is geographically and culturally, the more significant this becomes and the more the patient may start to wonder whether the physician has his or her best interests at heart and to whom the physician is ultimately accountable. If the third-party payor has elected for economic reasons to hire physicians who are physically located in another country instead of actually sitting in the intensive-care unit where the care is being given, who is to say that these physicians might not tailor the treatments to keep costs down so that they can keep their contracts, even if the outcomes weren't as good? This question of physician loyalty to third parties at the expense of patients, as discussed in chapter 4, is just as relevant to local physicians as it is to foreign ones. Unless the patient has forged a personal connection with the physician, based upon trust, this can become more of an issue and compromise the physician's ability to treat illness and sickness in addition to disease.

HOW THE HEALTH-CARE ENVIRONMENT INFLUENCES PHYSICIAN-PATIENT COMMUNICATION

One topic that seems rarely to arise in the conversation about how to improve the quality of health care in this country is the way in which the physical environment within which patients and physicians interact affects their relationship. This seems odd, considering what a strong effect one's surroundings exert upon the perceptions of what transpires within them. Candlelight dinners are much more romantic than those eaten under the harsh glare of fluorescent tube lighting, after all. So how do the clinic and hospital environment affect physician-patient interaction?

A lot, it turns out.

Consider the "hospital smell," a medley of sanitizers, chemicals, and bodily fluids that causes many people to experience a vague sense of dread, unease, and stress. This is not much different than the way the smell of the dentist's office sets you up mentally for the drill as soon as you open the door, whether you've come in for a cleaning or a root canal. Researchers have found that by scenting dentists' offices with orange essential oils, patients reported improved mood and less anxiety. Doing something similar in clinics and hospitals could yield a similar effect in reducing anxiety, which, as I mentioned earlier, can greatly hamper a person's ability to absorb and process information.[46]

The same holds true for ambient lighting and background noise. In 2005, one busy urban British general practice moved from its old quarters into a newly constructed building especially designed with larger clinic rooms, improved lighting, and better noise control. Patients at that practice reported that both their anxiety levels and the quality of their communication with their physicians were substantially improved in the new location, and they specifically noted the improvements in lighting, space, and décor.[47]

The configuration of the actual space in which the clinical visit takes place can also have a powerful influence on the quality of the communication between physician and patient. Clinic rooms that are arranged so that the physician does not have to avert her focus from the patient during the visit improve the amount of eye contact and the quality of nonverbal communication.[48]

The concept of channeling the positive influences that facilities design can bring into improving physician-patient communication extends to hospitals as well. Patient rooms that are specifically designed to facilitate unhurried and uninterrupted conversations between patient and physician wind up fostering that very communication. For example, this means furnishing rooms with sufficient chairs for physicians to use during rounds so that they can sit down and converse at eye level with patients, instead of towering over them in their pressed white coats while the patients try to stay modest in their shapeless and gaping jonnies. There also need to be dedicated meeting rooms where patients and their physician(s) can sit down and meet, especially when multiple specialists are involved in the care or when patients are in shared rooms.

Patient satisfaction is becoming one of the factors that determine reimbursement, and it also affects a hospital's ability to capture and maintain market share in an increasingly competitive marketplace. It is therefore important to point out that patient-satisfaction scores with regards to nurses, physicians, and services provided in the hospital are higher when the rooms are more esthetically attractive.[49]

In a 2013 article in *TheAtlantic.com*, Lindsay Abrams described how the cancer treatment center at Cedars-Sinai hospital in Los Angeles was reconstructed with special attention paid to lighting and color. The makeover required a lot of thought, as the cancer center was physically located underground, and in its old set-up evoked tomb-like associations, exactly the opposite message one would want to send cancer patients, or any others, for that matter. The changes resulted in higher patient- and worker-satisfaction scores. This is not surprising, as patients have reported that viewing nature reduces stress and pain.[50] At the other end of the spectrum is what is seen in many patients hospitalized in intensive-care units that run around the clock without changes in lighting or ambient noise who develop delirium and/or frank psychotic symptoms known as ICU psychosis.

As D. Kirk Hamilton and Robin Diane Orr of the Center for Health Design have written, health-care facility design sends a powerful message to patients, often even before they meet the physician(s) who will be caring for them:

> There are obvious differences between healthcare organizations whose buildings feature soaring lobbies full of plaques recognizing prominent donors, those whose pleasantly lit lobbies are filled with friendly welcoming faces, and those whose dim and dusty lobbies are simply vestibules leading to a bleak set of confusing corridors. The space in which patients are met and the actions of those they encounter begin to tell those patients how they will be perceived and how the organization might care for them.[51]

This is no mere abstraction but the subject of serious research dedicated to identifying evidence-based design, specifically in health care. And indeed, the Center for Health Design, founded in 1993, is one organization dedicated to this area. Its stated goal is to strive for "a world where every hospital, health clinic, treatment center, doctor's office, and residential care facility is designed to improve both the quality of care and outcomes for patients, residents, and staff."[52]

CLOSING THOUGHTS

In this chapter I've discussed some of what can be done at a systems level to improve communication between physicians and patients, and I have tried to show that the pursuit of lower health costs through increased physician throughput may easily achieve the opposite results. In the final chapter, I'll demonstrate how the physician-patient interaction can be improved upon when both patient and physician, individually, actively address many of the issues that I've brought up throughout the book, and I'll offer practical suggestions for both about how to do so. I'll also present a blueprint for revamping the clinical encounter, using HIT, so that its therapeutic effects can be extended far beyond the minutes patient and physician spend with each other, achieving better results and outcomes and improving overall efficiency.

8

PUTTING IT ALL TOGETHER

Creating a Better Clinical Encounter

Be more interested than afraid.

—Mitchell B. Rider, MD, as told to his daughter Elizabeth A. Rider, MSW, MD

IN THE final chapter of this book, I'll focus mostly on those things that individual patients and physicians can do to improve their interactions with one another. In doing so, I'll make a lot of use of the terms *medical encounter* and patient or physician *visit*. For the purposes of this discussion, *medical encounter* will describe the entire time spent by the patient within the medical system, from the moment he enters the clinic or hospital until the time he leaves. *Visit*, however, will refer only to that portion of the encounter during which the patient and the physician directly interact. Lots can be done to improve the quality of communication during the visit itself. However, because the visit is only one component of the medical encounter, by making the other portions of the encounter more useful and efficient, it is possible to improve the quality of the communication within the visit itself, especially by creating ample opportunity for key messages to be reinforced.

IMPROVING COMMUNICATION BEFORE THE ACTUAL VISIT

Sitting in the waiting room, especially when the physician is behind schedule, can be very frustrating. The chairs are uncomfortable, it is nearly impossible to escape the coughing and sneezing of others, and the magazines are generally just not that interesting. Waiting itself can also generate a lot of anxiety, especially when the purpose of the appointment is to go over test results. Unsurprisingly, the longer the wait times, the less satisfied patients are.[1]

It doesn't have to be that way. Instead of having patients just sit there and stew as the minutes tick by, the previsit time could be utilized for a variety of defined purposes, such as targeted information gathering and entry and patient education. Not only would this add value to the entire medical encounter, but it would also send a powerful message to patients that they and their time are valued and respected, which in turn would lead to increased satisfaction.[2]

For example, one group found that screening a twenty-three-minute video in the waiting room of a sexually transmitted diseases (STD) clinic promoting safe-sex practices led to an almost 10 percent reduction in the subsequent incidence of infections among those who had watched the video. Another group found that showing a six-minute video about STD to young women who had just been diagnosed with pelvic inflammatory disease—a complication of STD—resulted in a threefold increase in them bringing their sexual partners to be tested and treated.[3]

The use of informational videos about upcoming surgical procedures, either as a stand-alone modality or in addition to physician explanations, can significantly bolster patient knowledge and understanding about what they are about to undergo.[4] Not only does this reduce anxiety, but it also provides patients with valuable information about what they will need to do before and after the procedure, guidance about common complications, and instructions about when to seek additional medical attention in the event that things don't go as smoothly as planned. When shown before the physician visit, such educational videos can help patients identify points that need further clarification from the physician and encourage them to write down and ask their questions during the visit itself. When shown after the visit, they can reinforce the content that was discussed but that may not have been fully understood and/or absorbed.

Filling out forms prior to the visit is something most patients are accustomed to. Usually, the majority of the questions relate to demographics, insurance details, medications, and the past medical history. What patients are *not* routinely asked about, however, is what their agenda for the visit is. By this I don't just mean the disease-oriented chief complaints (headache, chest pain, fever, sore throat) but also those concerns related to illness and to sickness that might easily get forgotten during the visit itself. For example: *it's getting harder for me to get up from bed to the bathroom at night, and I'm worried that this means I'm going to have to move into a nursing home where I won't know anyone and be treated like an invalid; I need refills for three prescriptions, my medications are really expensive, and I'd like to be on less expensive ones if possible; I need a letter for the electric company so they don't shut off my power, leaving me unable to use my asthma machine if I get sick.*

Asking patients to sit down in advance of the visit—or, even better, before the encounter itself—and prepare an agenda such as this is not a trivial exercise. Detached from the pressures of the visit, it allows the patient an opportunity to identify calmly and articulate those issues that are of most concern to him. The very act of writing them down can embolden the patient to raise them with the physician and help him overcome what might be an initial reluctance to do so for some of the reasons discussed earlier, such as stigma, shame, or worry that his own parallel belief systems might be dismissed or even ridiculed by the physician. Referring to the list during the visit helps make sure that all of the important questions get asked and prevents the frustration of the patient remembering them only on the way back home. A lot of these questions, related though they are to the patient's medical condition and care, might otherwise not be addressed by the physician, simply because she is unaware of them (*does that "pulmonary nodule" on my son's chest X ray mean that he has cancer?*). The visit agenda can be entered into a dedicated portion of the previsit intake form and uploaded into the electronic health record (EHR) or brought into the physician immediately before the visit, to give the physician insight into the patient's mindset and concerns and to serve as a road map for the visit itself.

Another reason why preparing visit agendas is so important is because the majority of people now routinely research health questions on the Internet. A recent Pew survey of more than three thousand adults found that almost two-thirds seek out health information online, and more than one-third self-diagnose based upon this information.[5] Because so much online information is inaccurate, it often directly contradicts that provided by the physician, resulting in uncertainty, which in turn undermines the trust necessary for good treatment adherence.

Unfortunately, that survey also found that only 53 percent of the respondents had actually discussed their Internet-acquired information with their physicians. It is certainly true that many physicians find it challenging to deal with patients who've done research online and discourage talking about their findings with them for all sorts of reasons. However, I personally am grateful when patients talk to me about things they've heard or read elsewhere because it provides me with an opportunity to address their concerns, which, even though they may lack a scientific basis, are real enough to them. My own experience is that my patients are perfectly willing to trust me—this is, after all, why they come to see me in the first place—and once I explain to them, for example, why I truly believe that the MMR vaccine will *not* cause their child to become autistic, they are more than happy to follow my recommendations. I suspect that their responses would be altogether different if instead of respectfully addressing their concerns, I were to dismiss them by saying something like: *You really should know better than to believe all that nonsense you read online.*

ONE SCENARIO FOR USING HEALTH-INFORMATION TECHNOLOGY (HIT) TO IMPROVE THE MEDICAL ENCOUNTER

It is easy to imagine how the medical encounter could be greatly improved upon by incorporating the above and making use of the opportunities that HIT offers. Here is a hypothetical scenario in which this plays out. Upon arrival to the clinic, a patient would be checked in; the check-in process would include a screening to determine the patient's general and health literacy. The patient would then be given a tablet device, which she would use to update details of her recent medical history, any medication allergies, and to reconcile her current medication list with the one on file from her previous visit. Patients identified as having low general and/or health literacy or impaired cognitive faculties because of disease, medications, or other reasons would be provided with assistance by a trained clinical assistant or nurse. The patient would also have the ability to flag specific items or concerns for discussion with her physician and to type in questions that she might otherwise forget to bring up during the visit. She could then request refills for her prescriptions as needed and update her pharmacy information so that the scripts could be faxed over directly at the end of the visit. She would also be able to do the same for any forms she needed, such as for school or work.

After the process of information gathering was completed, the patient would be able to watch a series of short informational videos that had been specifically selected based upon her medical history, gender, and demographics, along with others of her choosing that were relevant to any specific health concerns she might have. These would be available in a variety of languages and might, for example, provide information about prevention and screening for conditions she might be at risk for or about the importance of getting the annual flu shot. After watching the videos, she could then go ahead and schedule appointments for these on the spot, with the tablet.

All the information that the patient had entered on the tablet would upload directly into the EHR and be accessible to the physician in real time during the visit via his computer. By reviewing the agenda items listed by the patient immediately before the actual visit, the physician would have a better understanding of the patient's concerns and be able to address them even if the patient herself neglected to bring them up during the visit. The physician would also be able to navigate the visit itself better, in accordance with this information. Likewise, because so much of the information necessary for the visit would already have been entered in advance, the physician could review it quickly, leaving more time to spend on those issues that were of greatest concern to the patient. One of the more frustrating things for any physician is to hear, as the patient is halfway out the door after most of the visit has spent discussing the patient's athlete's foot, is something along the lines of: *Oh, and by the way, doc? I've had this sore on my chest for the last three months that hasn't gotten any better, and in fact, seems to be getting bigger . . .*

At the end of the visit, the patient would return to the waiting room, where she could watch additional videos, selected by the physician, which would reinforce and elaborate upon what had just been discussed. Others would be queued up automatically by virtue of certain tests having been ordered or medications having been prescribed during the visit. These might include explanations about proper technique of medicine administration and storage, review of some of the possible side effects of newly prescribed medications, or perhaps provide an overview of some practical weight-loss strategies. If, for example, a colonoscopy had been ordered, the patient might watch a short video explaining how to prepare for it, what to expect from the procedure itself, and what the expected time frame might be for the results to return. If she didn't quite understand how many bottles of colon prep she would need to drink prior to the procedure, she could replay the video a second, third, or fourth time without feeling stupid or frustrated by wasting precious face time with the physician, time that might otherwise have been used to discuss other issues of importance to her. If she had additional questions beyond what the videos could explain, a nurse would be available to answer them as needed.

Before completing the medical encounter, a menu would allow the patient to select printouts about specific topics, which she could then take home for further review. These would be in addition to personalized ones prepared for her by the physician, such as asthma-action plans, and others automatically selected for her because of a new diagnosis, tests or diagnostic procedures that had been ordered, or newly prescribed medications. As would be the case with the videos, these handouts could be provided in a variety of languages, which would help those with poor English proficiency. The patient could also request that links to the videos be sent to her by e-mail for further review at home. She might use the tablet to schedule future appointments: regular follow-ups, flu shots, and testing that had been ordered by the physician during the visit. A list of appointments to be scheduled would populate a specific menu to prevent her from forgetting to do so, and she could select to receive e-mail, text, or phone reminders, and/or a printout of the schedule prior to going home; all this would also free up time for the administrative staff. The patient would also be able to provide feedback about the quality of the clinical encounter, including the visit itself, so that the overall patient experience within the clinic, practice, or hospital could be improved upon. Once everything was complete, she would return the tablet and leave.

Notice that in this scenario (parts of which are already playing out in different physician practices and settings) patient care is both more efficient *and* less hurried. The visit with the physician becomes only one part, albeit a very important one, of the continuum of care provided within the medical encounter and beyond. By eliminating those tasks currently done by physicians that don't actually need to be done by physicians, such as much of the data entry and patient education described above, physicians would have more time to spend on those tasks they are uniquely qualified to perform. Physicians would be able to probe much more deeply at the psychosocial aspects of illness and sickness and to reinforce the importance of good adherence and of preventive medicine. With patients assuming more responsibility for data entry into the medical record, physician workloads would be reduced, helping them care for larger panels of patients, something that would help mitigate the growing shortage of primary-care physicians.

Although integrating HIT into the clinical encounter like this would require an initial capital investment, it would also reduce work for the administrative staff. It is likely, too, that with the improved adherence, reduced medication errors, and higher rates of preventive medicine utilization that would result from the better use of physician time and the more comprehensive, non-physician-mediated education, patients would need to see, and be seen by, their physicians less frequently.

IMPROVING COMMUNICATION BETWEEN PHYSICIAN AND PATIENT DURING THE VISIT ITSELF

This next section comprises two parts: one intended primarily for patients, the other for physicians. However, this should not be taken to imply that patients cannot learn from the suggestions for physicians and vice versa. As a physician, I encourage my patients to follow the recommendations below because I find that when they do, our interactions become better and more satisfying. I hope that other physicians and medical professionals will share this experience and pass them along to their own patients as well.

The same is true for the suggestions aimed at physicians, which I believe are worthwhile for patients to read and reflect upon as well. One of the downsides of completing my medical training—even though sometimes it seemed as though it would never end!—is that I stopped receiving regular feedback on the quality of my work. Yet it's not as if the newly minted attending physician, just out of residency or fellowship, has learned all there is to know about how to communicate effectively with his patients. That certainly wasn't the case for me. I regret not receiving regular feedback from patients on my own interpersonal communication skills because I am sure that I would benefit from it greatly. For example, if someone were to say to me: *Gee, Dr. Rosen, you spent an awful lot of time typing on your computer but hardly seemed to pay attention when I was describing my son's cough to you,* you can be sure that I'd take it to heart. This is why I believe that the suggestions for physicians will be as useful for patients to read as they will be for physicians and other medical personnel. They are intended to encourage the nonphysician reader to embrace the notion that bad communication by their physicians should *not* be accepted as the inevitable cost of getting good medical care, which, as I've shown in the previous chapters, ultimately proves to be suboptimal. My hope is that these pointers will empower patients to insist upon better communication with their physicians, which will result in better health outcomes for themselves as well as yielding more satisfaction for all involved.

FOR THE PATIENT

Take charge of the visit. This is how you, as a patient, can improve the communication between you and your physician.

1. *Prepare an agenda ahead of time, including a list of questions you need answers to.* Make two copies, one for you and one for your physician, which you can give to her at the beginning of the visit, or better yet, just prior to it, so that she can do her best to tailor the visit to meet your needs. That way, you can both refer to the list and keep the visit on track. The questions should be both specific and general. Specific questions you can prepare in advance might relate to the concerns that brought you to see the physician in the first place. *I've noticed I've been getting short of breath climbing the stairs. Might this be because of any of the medications I'm currently taking? Do I need to have any testing done? If so, will it be painful?* General questions might be those that could come up in any visit. *What is the purpose of the new medication you're prescribing me? What are the potential side effects? How long will I need to take it for? Will it interact adversely with any of the other medications I'm currently on? I know that you remember that I am allergic to amoxicillin; should I be concerned about having an allergic reaction to this medication as well?* The Agency for Healthcare Research and Quality, for example, has lists of questions online available for patients to draw upon and use before, during, and after their visit with the physician.[6] There is also a question-building tool that patients can use to help formulate their own questions in advance of their visits.[7]

2. *Be honest and open about your concerns.* Your physician may be smart, but she's not a mind-reader, so don't expect her to guess what your problem is. If you've recently started to have painless rectal bleeding, *tell her about it*, and early enough in the visit so that you'll have plenty of time to discuss your concerns and to get the attention and the answers you need.

3. *Take notes.* Physicians have an annoying tendency to speak quickly and to lapse into jargon without warning. Most of us don't do this to show off and dazzle you with our knowledge; it's just that we have these conversations all the time, and what's jargon to laypeople is the language we think and conceptualize health, disease, illness, and sickness in. This makes it easy for us to forget that even though we may have said the same thing to three other people in just the last two days, it's still the first time *you're* hearing it and that it may be totally new for you. By taking notes, you force the physician to slow down his rapid-fire delivery, and you'll have more time to process what he's saying. This, in turn, can prompt you to ask clarifying questions. It will also help you keep track of the myriad instructions and suggestions that arise spontaneously and that won't necessarily be provided to you in a prepared handout at the end of the visit.

4. *Even better, bring someone else with you to the visit.* Your stress level going into the visit is higher than usual, even if you're not overtly aware of it, and it is very likely you aren't feeling at your best, either because of physical discomfort or because of the medications you're taking. All will take a toll on your concentration and make it more difficult for you to follow and keep track of what is being discussed, as well as making it harder to remember afterward. Bringing along a close family member or friend, especially one who can ask clarifying questions if you become overwhelmed and take notes for you, can be a big bonus when you try to recall exactly what was said.

5. *Make sure you know what medications (names and doses) you're on and the names of any you've had unusual or adverse reactions to in the past.* If you're seeing your primary-care physician, this information should already be in your chart, but reminding her of it can be very helpful to

prevent mix-ups and bad interactions between any new meds and those you're already on. This is especially important when she prescribes you a new medicine. It's worth remembering the study I mentioned in chapter 1 that found that patients who had mentioned their hypertension to their physicians were twice as likely to be treated for it as those who hadn't. Just because the information is written down somewhere in your record doesn't mean that it has permeated the physician's consciousness at that particular—and very important—moment. Physicians have lots of information to process, and it's vitally important that you make sure, before starting any new medication, that your physician has checked to see that you are not allergic to it or on something else that might negatively interact with the new medication.

Making sure of this is especially important with physicians you are meeting for the first time, in the emergency room, for example. They may have no access to any of this information beyond what you are able to tell them. Keeping a printed and up-to-date list of your current medications and drug allergies in your wallet or on a thumb drive can be life saving. It can help prevent confusion and is certainly much easier for physicians to work with than having to try to guess what you mean by "the little blue pill I take in the morning."

6. *When something isn't clear: speak up!* This visit is about you, and the physician is there to meet your needs. There is no such thing as a stupid question when it comes to your health and you don't understand what you're being told. Ask your questions, and ask them again, until you've received an answer that you understand and that satisfies you.

7. *Before the visit is over, make absolutely sure that you clearly understand what you are supposed to do* as far as treatment goes and under which circumstances you need to seek further medical care. As true for a routine office visit with your primary care physician as it is for a week-long stay in the hospital, these are the core reasons for the visit, after all. Unless you are sure that you understand the physician's treatment recommendations and what signs and symptoms indicate that the treatment isn't working, there is a much greater chance that something will go wrong. Being given a printed summary of the visit

containing this information can be very useful, but if the font is too small or the language opaque, you won't be able to rely upon it.

FOR THE PHYSICIAN

The physician has much more to think about and attend to insofar as improving the quality of her communication with her patients. The balance of power, knowledge, and experience is clearly in her favor. She is healthy; the patient is not. She is comfortable and secure within the familiar settings of her office; the patient is somewhere he'd much rather not be, anxious, uncomfortable, often half-naked. I've already discussed many of the surrounding issues (culture, bias, stigma, third-party intervention, disparate models of disease conceptualization, variability in illness behavior, and sickness) that strongly influence the interaction between physician and patient. To overcome most of these, the first step is to become aware that these obstacles, when present, even exist. The physician then needs to be open to learning about how these issues influence her own interactions with her patients. For example, this may include preemptively discussing uvulectomy (removal of the uvula) with Ethiopian-Jewish families ahead of their child's birth, to keep it from being carried out. Or it may entail developing more sensitivity to how obese patients perceive messages about the importance of weight loss and taking extra precautions to avoid coming across as insensitive or judgmental.

In this section, however, I'd like mostly to focus on practical steps that physicians can take each time they engage with their patients on a personal, one-to-one level. The first is to improve the quality of their nonverbal communication with their patients. In 1967, Albert Mehrabian and Susan Ferris published their seminal study showing that 93 percent of general interpersonal communication is nonverbal.[8] Although they constantly observe others, physicians are not always cognizant about what they themselves convey through their own body language and demeanor. That was the case with the nephrologist I described in chapter 7, who so terrified my patient without even realizing what was happening. In one study that explored physicians' nonverbal communication, patients identified forty-eight different types of nonverbal cues given by their physicians. These included: "tone of voice, eye-contact, facial expressions . . . exam room characteristics, touch, interpersonal distance, [physician dress], gestures, and posture."[9] The most commonly commented upon were tone of voice and eye contact.

Most medical students receive at least some training in basic communication skills. However, during the busy years of training and practice, when there always seems to be one more patient to see and one more discharge summary to sign, these can be neglected and then forgotten: there just never seems to be enough time. Concentrating on good communication skills becomes simply one more task that often winds up being relegated to a lower priority than other, more "important" ones, such as treating disease. As the physician Danielle Ofri writes in her book *What Doctors Feel*: "The medical student observes that even the most thoughtful and humanistic intern operates under the brutal calculus that every minute spent on nonessentials simply prolongs the work. Sure, it's wonderful to have an in-depth conversation with a patient . . . but none of these will get the work done."[10]

This, along with some of the psychological and emotional reasons for disengagement from patients which I discussed in chapter 5, can quickly become the norm for how the budding physician becomes accustomed to working. And although physician work-hours do improve once training is complete, the workload itself seems only to increase, making it difficult to change ingrained habits that seem otherwise to work just fine.

So here are a number of suggestions for physicians about how to better interact with their patients:

1. *Shake hands.* A handshake provides a formal beginning to the visit, transforming it from a chance meeting into a purposeful one. The handshake also provides both physician and patient with an opportunity to focus on the other fully and to connect nonverbally. In some

cultures, men and women who are not married to each other do not shake hands. Because I am accustomed to starting off my visits with a handshake, when this is not possible for cultural reasons, it can feel like the visit is starting off on the wrong foot. One solution I've found that works reasonably well is simply to wave hello to the patient from a distance of a few feet. Likewise, shaking hands at the end of the visit "seals the deal," providing a nonverbal commitment of both patient and physician to the success of the treatment plan that was just developed and agreed upon.

2. *Smile.* Whenever I come out of the operating room after doing a bronchoscopy I try to smile as broadly as possible while walking toward the parents. My first words after reintroducing myself are something like *Tommy is doing great,* even before shaking their hands, usually because I start speaking before I'm close enough to actually make physical contact. This defuses a lot of stress and, because it's true, serves as important reassurance even when the findings of the procedure itself are not as good as had been hoped for. Smiling at the beginning of the visit, regardless of where it takes place, is important because it dispels any notion on the part of your patient that you'd rather be doing something else, and it reinforces the message to the patient that you are there for him and eager to help. This is true even when the subject of the conversation is a difficult or disturbing one; when that comes up, the body language, including facial expressions, will change in accordance.

3. *Maintain eye contact as much as possible.* This is pretty straightforward. As an anonymous patient once told an interviewer: "you can feel [the personal attention by] how someone looks into your eyes, not making any notes or writing on a computer at that time; I can see the interest."[11]

4. *Sit, don't stand.* Sitting down projects focus and attention and sends the message that you're there intentionally for the patient and not just making a quick detour while on your way to something more important. Many patients feel that their physicians spend more time with them and are more attentive to their needs when seated.[12] Where

the physician sits relative to the patient is also important. In the inpatient setting, for example, it is much more respectful to be seated at eye level, or even a bit lower, as opposed to towering over the scantily clad patient, literally talking down to him.

5. Body position: Make sure to face the patient squarely, leaning forward and/or striking a relaxed body position. The patient needs to be the center of attention, not the computer or the attending on rounds. I've seen medical students presenting patients to their supervising physicians *with their backs to the patient!* It would be one thing if the object of discussion happened to be a statue or some other inanimate object, but it certainly is not OK to talk about someone behind your back in front of their face. That is disrespectful and demeaning and can also provoke a lot of unnecessary anxiety in the patient.

6. *Ask lots of open-ended questions throughout the visit.* Begin with questions such as *how can I help you?*, and conclude with *do you have any other questions?* Allowing the patient to frame her concerns in ways that make sense to her and to contextualize them in ways that may not be immediately intuitive to you is important if you want her, in turn, to understand what you are going to tell her regarding the disease and the treatment for it you will propose. It is also an important part of motivational interviewing, which I discussed in chapter 7.

7. *Let the patient state the agenda for the visit in his own words.* As pediatric subspecialist, I am often sent copies of a child's medical record in advance of the visit that I review ahead of time. After the initial introductions, I will often start the visit by saying something like: *Dr. Jones sent me over a lot of information about Simon, which I've already read through, and I understand that he's been hospitalized three times this winter because of pneumonia. But I'd like to hear from you about why you're here today, and how I can help you.* This serves many purposes: it reassures them that I care enough about their child to have taken the time to learn about him, and it also allows the parents to express in their own words what *they* are most concerned about, which may be completely different from what I understood from Dr. Jones's note. While there is usually good overlap between the concerns of the family and the referring

physician, this is not always the case. Occasionally there is enough of a discrepancy between what I've read and what I hear from the parents to make me rethink my initial assessment about what might be wrong with the child. In addition, asking the family to explain their concerns to me directly often provides a window through which I am able to learn about other underlying concerns that I might be able to allay or resolve with reassurance or with simple testing and that might otherwise not have come up: *A woman I work with has a cousin with cystic fibrosis, and I'm really nervous that that's what this is, even though the pediatrician has been telling me that my son only has asthma.*

8. *Follow up on the patient's questions by asking him whether he has any additional concerns or questions.* I have often found that many patients and/or their parents will start off by asking a very innocuous and straightforward question, almost as if they're testing me to gauge my response. The next question, however, is usually the one they're much more concerned about. It is usually prefaced by something like *I know this is the crazy mom talking . . .* and then leads into something they've heard from a friend or read about on the Internet: *. . . but are these meds going to harm my child's brain development?* I really like being asked this kind of question because it shows me that I've established enough trust with the patient or his parent and that they're not concerned that I might mock them or make them feel foolish.

9. *Respect silences, and use them strategically.* Silences embedded within conversations, especially about the weighty topics that are usually discussed between physicians and patients, should not be seen as vacuums that need to be rushed into and filled. Very often, these silences occur because the patient is processing what you've just told her. Talking over these silences often achieves the opposite effect, overwhelming the patient with additional information as she is still grappling with what you told her thirty seconds ago. Respect these natural breaks in the conversation, and use them to take stock of where the patient is emotionally. If the patient is too anxious or upset, redirect the conversation until you sense that you can proceed with what you feel still needs to be discussed

10. *Be sensitive to emotions, your own as well as the patient's.* With experience comes an appreciation of what a "typical" response to a diagnosis or bad news is, within the context of cultural differences, and what is not. When a patient responds in an unexpected way to something you've said, it may be because there are other concerns underlying the ones you might be addressing that may be more important to him than you appreciate. This was what happened to me with Sally's mother. An unusual response on the part of your patient may also arise because you've misread him and approached the issue with a style inappropriate for that particular patient, even though it may work well enough for most others. In either case, pointing that out nonjudgmentally and simply asking what the matter is can be very effective in getting the conversation back on track: *I notice that you're really upset right now. What is it that's upsetting you so much right now?* If it turns out that something you said came across as insensitive, it is often best simply to apologize and even ask to "take it back."

It is true that some patients simply rub us the wrong way, and vice versa. Transference and countertransference occur frequently within interpersonal relationships, including that between physician and patient. The physician and psychoanalyst Michael Balint, who dedicated much of his professional life to understanding and improving the interaction between the general practitioner and patient, viewed this as one of the more important aspects of the physician-patient relationship.[13] Because, however, the whole purpose of the visit is to address the needs of the patient, not those of the physician, it is important for the physician to identify feelings of anger, humiliation, revulsion, or disdain as they arise within him so that they can be recognized for what they are, their source identified, and the emotions defused. Often they are caused by resentment and a sense of insult bred by a feeling of being disrespected. Recognizing them for what they are and consciously choosing to set them aside so as to focus on the real issue—the well-being of the patient—may be necessary to get the visit back on track.

This can happen, for example, when caring for an asthmatic child who keeps getting sick and whose mother doesn't give him the medications he's been prescribed. It can certainly be tempting to think: *If she doesn't bother to make sure that her kid takes his meds, of course he's going to get sick! Why is she wasting my time like this?* Yet the fundamental truth is that that mother is back in my office, missing half a day of work and pulling her kid out of school, which tells me that she is genuinely concerned about her child's health, even though she doesn't seem to be able to get the meds into him. Perhaps the issue is the cost of the medications themselves, but she's too embarrassed to say so.

It can also occur, for example, when caring for a patient who continues to smoke even after having had a heart attack. His doing so, despite having been told by you and others that he needs to quit, need not be construed as a repudiation of you and everything you stand for. Ultimately, your role as physician is not to dress the patient down or to shame him but to help him stay as healthy as possible, within the confines of what you have to work with. Getting angry at him may give you momentary satisfaction but may also serve to push him away and prevent you from making headway in treating some of his other risk factors for cardiac disease such as high cholesterol and hypertension.

11. *Avoid jargon and technical language as much as possible.* Health-literacy disparities are much more prevalent than most of us appreciate. The need to explain medical concepts in lay terms is as true for a patient who happens to be a medical professional as it for one who didn't complete high school, because of the ways in which anxiety and discomfort can affect a patient's cognitive faculties. Punctuate your explanations by regularly asking: *do you have any questions?* or *does that make sense?* If patients wants more detailed explanations, they'll ask you for them, but the opposite is not always true, either because of shame or because they're simply too overwhelmed and nothing you're saying is registering anymore.

12. *Use pictures to your advantage.* Pictures can help transform abstract concepts that may be terrifying to the uninitiated into tangible realities that may be much easier for your patients to grasp.

I was recently asked to consult on a five-year-old child in one of the intensive-care units who had been admitted because of severe pneumonia. The purpose of the consult was to see if there was any work-up that needed to be done to identify a possible underlying problem which might have predisposed the child to getting so sick to begin with. In terms of the boy's acute needs, he was actually doing better than he had been, and, in fact, he had just been weaned from the ventilator earlier that morning after being on it for the last three days.

After reviewing the child's chart and films, I went into the room and introduced myself to the parents, who were both disheveled and looked as though they hadn't slept in over a week. They were beside themselves with worry over their son who, until one week earlier, had "never been sick." The child was breathing quickly when I saw him and didn't have much appetite. Although off the ventilator, he continued to require supplemental oxygen via nasal cannula.

The parents and I spoke, following which I examined their son. Afterward, I told them that it looked like he was making good progress, based upon my examination and everything I had learned from his chart. They both nodded their heads wearily, their faces showing just how hard the events of the last few days had been for them.

I then asked whether either of them had gone home since he had been admitted. They both shook their heads. Because the worst seemed to be behind them, I urged them to go home, separately, for a few hours each at a time. I felt that it was really important for their own mental health to leave the dimly lit ICU room, with its constantly beeping monitors and equipment, so that they could shower and get a few hours of sleep in their own bed. However, even though both parents were nodding their heads, it seemed that nothing I had just said had registered.

"Have you seen today's chest X ray?" I asked.

No, they had not.

We stepped outside the room, and I pulled up the X ray on the computer terminal, alongside one that had been taken two days earlier. The interval improvement between the two was striking. Despite not having any medical background and never having looked critically at a chest X ray before, once I oriented them to the images they could clearly see the differences between them.

The next afternoon I came by to check in on the child, who was now sitting up in bed, off oxygen, and watching TV. He looked great. The father, clean-shaven today, was asleep on the sofa-bed by the window. I chose not to disturb him. As for the child's mother, his nurse told me she had gone home earlier that day for the first time since he had been admitted.

13. *Make use of medical decision-making aids with your patients to engage and involve them in directing their own care.* These can be in whichever format works best for their individual learning style: text, picture, video, or audio. They can, and should, be used at any time before, during, or after the visit, as discussed earlier.

14. *Provide your patients with handouts and customized instruction sheets that they can refer back to.* Not only will this improve outcomes when they realize that they've forgotten what exactly they are supposed to do, but they will also save you and your office staff time by reducing the number of phone calls for clarification.

15. *Be available.* Make sure there are mechanisms in place for questions to be answered in a timely manner, whether by you personally, a nurse, or other office staff. This can be done by telephone, e-mail, or any other medium approved by your practice. My own impression is that the more patients understand how to reach you if and when a problem arises and know that you or someone working with you will respond quickly, the less likely they are to take advantage of that for frivolous matters.

16. *Be honest.* Don't promise miracles, and don't pretend to know what you don't, but by the same token, don't hold back on information you've gleaned from your years of experience. True: you may not have all the answers. You are only human after all, but you do possess the knowledge and understanding that your patients desperately need and seek. Likewise, if a medical error has occurred, be open about it with both the patient and the family, and apologize for the negative outcome that arose from it, within the context of your institution's policy. The topic of the medical apology is beyond the scope of this book, but it is becoming more and more accepted within the American healthcare system.[14]

17. *Above all, be compassionate and empathetic.* Or as my father used to tell me as a child: be a *mensch*.

A colleague of mine who works in primary care recently told me about an interaction she had just had with one of the medical students rotating through her clinic. After spending the afternoon observing some of the other providers, she met with the student to ask him how his day was.

"Not so great," he responded dismissively. "There were a lot of patients, but they all turned out to have nothing."

Wow, she thought, and sat down to have a long conversation with him about what he meant by "nothing." No one takes half a day off from work, pulls their kid out of school, pays a co-pay, and sits in a crowded waiting room with lots of other sick and miserable kids for "nothing." The problem that brings people in can be one of disease, which both physician and patient recognize; one of illness without disease, perceived subjectively by the patient but not by the physician; or entirely psychosocial in nature. Irrespective of its etiology, however, the problem is real enough to the patient, and solving, rather than dismissing, is something the physician should strive to do, irrespective of its etiology.

I learned this lesson early on in my residency in Israel, with two different kids whom I saw on the same night. One was a six-day-old girl, brought in by her mother because "her breathing didn't seem right." The senior resident had examined her, found her to be fine, and wanted to send the baby and her mother home after a few hours of observation. The mother refused to leave, however, insisting that something was simply not "right" with the infant—her fifth. I asked him what he was going to do with them, and he told me that he planned to let the mother stay in the emergency room for as long as she wanted to until she was ready to go. He did not, however, intend to admit her to the ward, so she camped out overnight in one of the smaller rooms, dozing in a chair next to her baby's crib. However, when she still refused to leave the next morning, the day team admitted her.

Poking my head into the room over the course of that night, I felt somewhat disdainful of the mother, who seemed to fit the bill of the overanxious parent. It was only later that I learned that this mother had no help with her children other than her husband, who had resumed studying at his *yeshiva* the day after the infant had been born. The combination of stress, physical fatigue, and sleeplessness had brought the mother to a point near collapse, and she was simply unable to continue caring for her children or for herself unassisted. I was ashamed of how callously I had felt toward her and was very pleased when I heard that the social worker was able to arrange for her and her baby to transfer out of the hospital into respite care.

The second child I saw that night was a ten-week-old boy who was brought in by his father a little after three in the morning. I was standing behind the counter chatting with one of the nurses, the waiting room having finally emptied out, when he came in.

"Doctor," he said anxiously, "I've discovered a lump in my son's chest."

I walked him into one of the exam rooms and asked him to undress his son so that I could see what it was he was worried about. As he unwrapped the child from the blanket he was swaddled in, I could easily see the boy's xiphoid process, the triangular-shaped bone at the base of the sternum, angled a bit more prominently upward than usual, but nothing worrisome from a medical perspective.

"This?" I asked, touching it as it undulated with each breath the now fully awake infant drew, beginning to smile as I wondered how it was, exactly, that it had taken this man this long to notice what his son's chest looked like in the almost three months that had passed since he was born.

"Yes," he answered, looking up from where my finger was resting to look at me. He, too, began to smile.

"Doctor," he said, "I don't know what this is, but from your smile I can tell that it isn't serious, and that's good enough for me."

After I explained to him that it was a normal anatomic variant and nothing to worry about, the father thanked me, shook my hand, bundled his baby up, and went home. Nothing to worry about, perhaps, but certainly not "nothing" to this father at three in the morning. Likewise with the newborn girl whose mother was on the verge of collapse. As my department chief Dr. Sinai would repeatedly tell us in her often blunt manner whenever she saw anyone overly focused on a patient's disease at the exclusion of her other needs, "Any idiot can prescribe antibiotics to treat an ear infection, but that's not what makes you a good physician."

CLOSING THOUGHTS AND SUMMARY

I began this book by describing the importance of good physician-patient communication to the healing process and by discussing some of the forces, primarily economic, that threaten its quality. I then discussed some of the cultural and contextual factors that can influence and often impede this communication. Exploring the concept of illness—which in the vast majority of cases is *the* reason patients come to see physicians in the first place—as distinct from disease, I've tried to show how important it is for physicians to expand their clinical focus to include illness as well as disease. By probing at those aspects of illness that are most troubling to the patient—through motivational interviewing, for example—the physician may well be able to find ways to transform illness behavior, specifically in ways that improve adherence. Likewise, by pointing out that even though it may appear that only the patient and physician are present in the clinic or exam room, the presence of other forces and entities (government, third-party payors) keenly influences their interaction in all that relates to stigma, bias, and sick roles as determined by society. Without recognizing their presence, their influence may be stronger than that of the physician herself, whether or not either patient or physician is aware of them. Finally, I have discussed the influence of external and health-care systemic factors on communication between physicians and patients and tried to provide guidance on ways in which individual physicians and patients each can work at improving this communication, in ways that will serve both *and* benefit society.

I hope that I have succeeded in convincing you that by actively nurturing and cultivating the very basis of the physician-patient relationship, namely, the communication that exists between the two, health outcomes can be improved, costs can be reduced, and both patient and physician satisfaction can increase. This is, after all, an issue that does or will affect each and every one of us. It is vitally important that we preserve and work actively to enhance the quality of our relationships and interactions with our physicians. We must not allow the quality of our health care to be determined solely by so-called efficiency experts whose misguided focus on short-term profits and savings may lead to the undermining and degradation of the care available to us in our hour of need.

We all deserve better.

NOTES

1. BETTER OUTCOMES, LOWER COSTS

1. A. B. Martin et al., "Growth in US Health Spending Remained Slow in 2010: Health Share of Gross Domestic Product Was Unchanged from 2009," *Health Affairs* 31 (2012): 208–219.
2. http://resources.iom.edu/widgets/vsrt/healthcare-waste.html.
3. Bonnie Blair O'Connor, foreword to Chloë Atkins, *My Imaginary Illness: A Journey Into Uncertainty and Prejudice in Medical Diagnosis* (Ithaca, N.Y.: Cornell University Press, 2010), xii.
4. Michael Balint, *The Doctor, His Patient, and the Illness*, 4th ed. (New York: International Universities Press, 1974), 116.
5. American Board of Medical Specialties, "Facts About the 2008 ABMS Consumer Survey: How Americans Choose Their Doctors," http://www.abms.org/News_and_Events/Media_Newsroom/pdf/ABMS_Survey_Fact_Sheet.pdf.
6. Kathy Davis, Cathy Shoen, and Kristof Streikis, "Mirror, Mirror on the Wall: How the Performance of the U.S. Health Care System Compares Internationally," 2010 update, The Commonwealth Fund, June 2010, http://www.commonwealthfund.org/~/media/Files/Publications/Fund%20Report/2010/Jun/1400_Davis_Mirror_Mirror_on_the_wall_2010.pdf.
7. S. P. Deshpande and J. DeMello, "An Empirical Investigation of Factors Influencing Career Satisfaction of Primary Care Physicians," *Journal of the American Board of Family Medicine* 23 (2010): 762–769.
8. M. A. Stewart, "Effective Physician-Patient Communication and Health Outcomes: A Review," *Canadian Medical Association Journal* 152 (1995): 1423–1433.
9. L. Paley et al., "Utility of Clinical Examination in the Diagnosis of Emergency Department Patients Admitted to the Department of Medicine of an Academic Hospital," *Archives of Internal Medicine* 171, no. 15 (August 2011): 1394–1396.

10. R. R. Khanna et al., "Missed Opportunities for Treatment of Uncontrolled Hypertension at Physician Office Visits in the United States, 2005 Through 2009," *Archives of Internal Medicine* 172 (2012): 1344–1345.

11. R. T. Zweigoron, H. J. Binns, and R. R. Tanz, "Unfilled Prescriptions in Pediatric Primary Care," *Pediatrics* 130 (2012): 620–626; A. S. Adams et al., "Health System Factors and Antihypertensive Adherence in a Racially and Ethnically Diverse Cohort of New Users," *Archives of Internal Medicine* 172 (2012): 1–8.

12. J. A. Cramer et al., "Medication Compliance and Persistence: Terminology and Definitions," *Value Health* 11, no. 1 (January–February 2008): 44–47.

13. K. Rost, "The Influence of Patient Participation on Satisfaction and Compliance," *Diabetes Education* 15 (1989): 139–143; Y. Liu et al., "Adherence to Adjuvant Hormone Therapy in Low-Income Women with Breast Cancer: The Role of Provider-Patient Communication," *Breast Cancer Research and Treat*ment (December 2012), PMID: 23263740; F. Mostashari et al., "Acceptance and Adherence with Antiretroviral Therapy Among HIV-Infected Women in a Correctional Facility," *Journal of Acquired Immune Deficiency Syndrome and Human Retrovirology* 18, no. 4 (August 1998): 341–348.

14. R. Kumar et al., "Decision-Making Role Preferences Among Patients with HIV: Associations with Patient and Provider Characteristics and Communication Behaviors," *Journal of General Internal Medicine* 25 (2010): 517–523; C. Haywood Jr. et al., "The Association of Provider Communication with Trust Among Adults with Sickle Cell Disease," *Journal of General Internal Medicine* 25 (2010): 543–548; C. Haywood Jr. et al., "Hospital Self-Discharge Among Adults with Sickle-Cell Disease (SCD): Associations with Trust and Interpersonal Experiences with Care," *Journal of Hospital Medicine* 5 (2010): 289–294.

15. H. Craig and B. Wright, "Nonadherence to Prophylactic Medication: Negative Attitudes Toward Doctors a Strong Predictor," *Australian Family Physician* 41, no. 10 (October 2012): 815–818.

16. D. C. Bultman and B. L. Svarstad, "Effects of Physician Communication Style on Client Medication Beliefs and Adherence with Antidepressant Treatment," *Patient Education and Counseling* 40 (2000): 173–185; R. Tamblyn et al., "Influence of Physicians' Management and Communication Ability on Patients' Persistence with Antihypertensive Medication," *Archives of Internal Medicine* 170, no. 12 (June 2010): 1064–1072; D. Schillinger et al., "Closing the Loop: Physician Communication with Diabetic Patients Who Have Low Health Literacy," *Archives of Internal Medicine* 163, no. 1 (2003): 83–90.

17. V. Francis, B. M. Korsch, and M. J. Morris, "Gaps in Doctor-Patient Communication: Patients' Response to Medical Advice," *New England Journal of Medicine* 280 (1969): 535–540; C. Haywood Jr. et al., "Examining the Characteristics and Beliefs of Hydroxyurea Users and Nonusers Among Adults with Sickle Cell Disease," *American Journal of Hematology* 86 (2011): 85–87.

18. N. K. Choudhry et al. "Post-Myocardial Infarction Free Rx Event and Economic Evaluation (MI FREEE) Trial: Full Coverage for Preventive Medications After Myocardial Infarction," *New England Journal of Medicine* 365, no. 22 (December 2011): 2088–2097.

19. I. B. Wilson et al., "Physician-Patient Communication About Prescription Medication Nonadherence: A Fifty-State Study of America's Seniors," *Journal of General Internal Medicine* 22, no. 1 (January 2007): 6–12.

20. B. A. Briesacher et al., "Comparison of Drug Adherence Rates Among Patients with Seven Different Medical Conditions," *Pharmacotherapy* 28 (2008): 437–443.

21. L. Osterberg and T. Blaschke, "Adherence to Medication," *New England Journal of Medicine* 353, no. 5 (August 2005): 487–497.

22. J. E. Bailey et al., "Antihypertensive Medication Adherence, Ambulatory Visits, and Risk of Stroke and Death," *Journal of General Internal Medicine* 25, no. 6 (June 2010): 495–503; H. B. Bosworth et al., "Medication Adherence: A Call for Action," *American Heart Journal* 162 (2011): 412–424.

23. J. E. Bailey et al., "Risk Factors Associated with Antihypertensive Medication Nonadherence in a Statewide Medicaid Population," *American Journal of Medical Science* (August 2012), PMID: 22885626; Steven Machlin and Sadeq Chowdhury, "Expenses and Characteristics of Physician Visits in Different Ambulatory Care Settings, 2008," Medical Expenditure Panel Survey, Agency for Healthcare Research and Quality, statistical brief 318, March 2011, http://meps.ahrq.gov/data_files/publications/st318/stat318.pdf; E. Stranges, N. Kowlessar, and A. Elixhauser, "Components of Growth in Inpatient Hospital Costs, 1997–2009," Healthcare Cost and Utilization Project, Agency for Healthcare Research and Quality, statistical brief 123, November 2011, http://www.hcup-us.ahrq.gov/reports/statbriefs/sb123.jsp; K. Nasseh et al., "Cost of Medication Nonadherence Associated with Diabetes, Hypertension, and Dyslipidemia," *American Journal of Pharmacy Benefits* 4 (2012): 41–47.

24. L. P. Ormerod, "Multidrug-Resistant Tuberculosis (MDR-TB): Epidemiology, Prevention, and Treatment," *British Medical Bulletin* 73–74 (June 2005): 17–24; Alison Bickford, "Twin Epidemics of Multidrug-Resistant Tuberculosis: Russia and New York City," *Virtual Mentor: Ethics Journal of the American Medical Association* 8, no. 4 (April 2006): 251–255.

25. D. M. Tarn et al., "Provider Views About Responsibility for Medication Adherence and Content of Physician-Older Patient Discussions," *Journal of the American Geriatrics Society* 60, no. 6 (June 2012): 1019–1026.

26. D. Noonan, Y. Jiang, and S. A. Duffy, "Utility of Biochemical Verification of Tobacco Cessation in the Department of Veterans Affairs," *Addict Behavior* 38, no. 3 (November 2012): 1792–1795; D. Shipton et al., "Reliability of Self-Reported Smoking Status by Pregnant Women for Estimating Smoking Prevalence: A Retrospective, Cross Sectional Study," *BMJ* 339 (October 2009): b4347.

27. Eric Topol, *The Creative Destruction of Medicine* (New York: Basic Books, 2012), 24.

28. E. R. Chasens et al., "Effect of Poor Sleep Quality and Excessive Daytime Sleepiness on Factors Associated with Diabetes Self-Management," *Diabetes Education* (November 2012); E. A. Beverly et al., "Look Who's (Not) Talking: Diabetic Patients' Willingness to Discuss Self-Care with Physicians," *Diabetes Care* 35, no. 7 (2012): 1466–1472; G. van Servellen et al., "Individual and System Level Factors Associated with Treatment Nonadherence

in Human Immunodeficiency Virus–Infected Men and Women," *AIDS Patient Care STDS* 16, no. 6 (June 2002): 269–281.

29. C. Skott, "Expressive Metaphors in Cancer Narratives," *Cancer Nursing* 25 (2002): 230–235.

30. Bultman and Svarstad, "Effects of Physician Communication Style."

31. http://www.cancer.gov/cancertopics/types/commoncancers.

32. A. J. Forster et al., "The Incidence and Severity of Adverse Events Affecting Patients After Discharge from the Hospital," *Annals of Internal Medicine* 138, no. 3 (February 2003): 161–167; J. Brock et al. (Care Transitions Project Team), "Association Between Quality Improvement for Care Transitions in Communities and Rehospitalizations Among Medicare Beneficiaries," *Journal of the American Medical Association* 309, no. 4 (January 2013): 381–391; S. F. Jencks, M. V. Williams, and E. A. Coleman, "Rehospitalizations Among Patients in the Medicare Fee-for-Service Program," *New England Journal of Medicine* 360 (2009): 1418–1428; Center for Medicare and Medicaid Services, Readmissions Reduction Program, http://www.cms.gov/Medicare/Medicare-Fee-for-Service-Payment/AcuteInpatientPPS/Readmissions-Reduction-Program.html.

33. Forster et al., "The Incidence and Severity of Adverse Events."

34. A. N. Makaryus and E. A. Friedman, "Patients' Understanding of Their Treatment Plans and Diagnosis at Discharge," *Mayo Clinic Proceedings* 80 (2005): 991–994.

35. A. N. Makaryus and E. A. Friedman, "Does Your Patient Know Your Name? An Approach to Enhancing Patients' Awareness of Their Caretaker's Name," *Journal of Healthcare Quality* 27, no. 4 (July–August 2005): 53–56.

36. S. Kripalani et al., "Health Literacy and the Quality of Physician-Patient Communication During Hospitalization," *Journal of Hospital Medicine* 5, no. 5 (May–June 2010): 269–275.

37. D. R. Calkins et al., "Patient-Physician Communication at Hospital Discharge and Patients' Understanding of the Postdischarge Treatment Plan," *Archives of Internal Medicine* 157, no. 9 (May 1997): 1026–1030.

38. Jencks, Williams, and Coleman, "Rehospitalizations Among Patients in the Medicare Fee-for-Service Program."

39. A. A. Vashi et al., "Use of Hospital-Based Acute Care Among Patients Recently Discharged from the Hospital," *Journal of the American Medical Association* 309, no. 4 (2013): 364–371.

40. C. C. Wee, E. P. McCarthy, and R. S. Phillips, "Factors Associated with Colon Cancer Screening: The Role of Patient Factors and Physician Counseling," *Preventive Medicine* 41, no. 1 (July 2005): 23–29; S. A. Fox and J. A. Stein, "The Effect of Physician-Patient Communication on Mammography Utilization by Different Ethnic Groups," *Medical Care* 29 (1991): 1065–1081; A. N. Meguerditchian et al., "Do Physician Communication Skills Influence Screening Mammography Utilization?" *BMC Health Services Research* 12 (July 2012): 219.

41. A. F. Dempsey et al., "Alternative Vaccination Schedule Preferences Among Parents of Young Children," *Pediatrics* 128, no. 5 (2011): 848–856.

42. W. A. Orenstein, P. M. Strebel, and A. R. Hinman, "Building an Immunity Fence Against Measles," *Journal of Infectious Diseases* 196, no. 10 (November 2007): 1433–1453.

43. http://www.miller-mccune.com/science-environment/storks-vaccines-and-causation -10195.

44. P. Cockman et al., "Improving MMR Vaccination Rates: Herd Immunity Is a Realistic Goal," *BMJ* 343 (October 2011): d5703; Health Protection Agency (Britain), Deaths by Age Group: 1980–2008 (ONS data): Measles deaths—England and Wales, by Age Group, 1980–2008, http://www.hpa.org.uk/web/HPAweb&HPAwebStandard /HPAweb_C/1195733811885.

45. A. Kennedy, M. Basket, and K. Sheedy, "Vaccine Attitudes, Concerns, and Information Sources Reported by Parents of Young Children: Results from the 2009 Health Styles Survey," *Pediatrics* 127, suppl. 1 (May 2011): S92–99.

46. Paul Bignell, "Italian Court Reignites MMR Vaccine Debate After Award Over Child with Autism," *Independent* (June 17, 2012), http://www.independent.co.uk/life-style /health-and-families/health-news/italian-court-reignites-mmr-vaccine-debate-after -award-over-child-with-autism-7858596.html.

47. G. Bartlett et al., "Impact of Patient Communication Problems on the Risk of Preventable Adverse Events in Acute Care Settings," *Canadian Medical Association Journal* 178, no. 12 (June 2008): 1555–1562.

48. R. M. Epstein et al., "Patient-Centered Communication and Diagnostic Testing," *Annals of Family Medicine* 3 (2005): 415–421.

49. R. Chou et al., Clinical Guidelines Committee of the American College of Physicians, "Diagnostic Imaging for Low Back Pain: Advice for High-Value Health Care from the American College of Physicians," *Annals of Internal Medicine* 154 (2011): 181–189.

50. S. V. Srinivas, R. A. Deyo, and Z. D. Berger, "Application of 'Less Is More' to Low Back Pain," *Archives of Internal Medicine* 172 (2012): 1016–1020.

51. J. J. Fenton et al., "The Cost of Satisfaction: A National Study of Patient Satisfaction, Health Care Utilization, Expenditures, and Mortality," *Archives of Internal Medicine* 172, no. 5 (March 2012): 405–411.

52. B. E. Sirovich, S. Woloshin, and L. M. Schwartz, "Too Little? Too Much? Primary Care Physicians' Views on US Health Care: A Brief Report," *Archives of Internal Medicine* 171, no. 17 (September 2011): 1582–1585.

53. T. D. Shanafelt et al., "Burnout and Satisfaction with Work-Life Balance Among US Physicians Relative to the General US Population," *Archives of Internal Medicine* 172, no. 18 (2012): 1377–1385; http://www.medscape.com/features/slideshow/compensation/2012 /public; http://www.ncnp.org/journal-of-medicine/1250-survey-55-of-physicians-wouldnt -recommend-medicine-as-career-to-children.html.

54. J. R. B. Halbesleben and C. Rathert, "Linking Physician Burnout and Patient Outcomes: Exploring the Dyadic Relationship Between Physicians and Patients," *Health Care Management Review* 33 (2008): 29–39; J. DeVoe J et al., "Does Career Dissatisfaction Affect the Ability of Family Physicians to Deliver High-Quality Patient Care?" *Journal of Family Practice* 51 (2002): 223–228; R. Tamblyn et al., "Physician Scores on a National Clinical Skills Examination as Predictors of Complaints to Medical Regulatory Authorities," *Journal of the American Medical Association* 298, no. 9 (September 2007): 993–1001; W. Levinson

et al., "Physician Patient Communication: The Relationship with Malpractice Claims Among Primary Care Physicians and Surgeons," *Journal of the American Medical Association* 277, no. 7 (1997): 553–559; S. A. Seabury et al., "On Average, Physicians Spend Nearly 11 Percent of Their Forty-Year Careers with an Open, Unresolved Malpractice Claim," *Health Affairs* 32, no. 1 (January 2013): 111–119.

55. J. D. Waldman et al., "The Shocking Cost of Turnover in Health Care," *Health Care Management Review* 29 (2004): 2–7; 2011 American Medical Group Association and Cejka Search, *Physician Retention Survey* (Alexandria, Va.: American Medical Group Association, 2012).

2. ONE SIZE DOES *NOT* FIT ALL

1. Personal communication.

2. P. A. Ubel, A. M. Angott, and B. J. Zikmund-Fisher, "Physicians Recommend Different Treatments for Patients Than They Would Choose for Themselves," *Archives of Internal Medicine* 171, no. 7 (2011): 630–634.

3. Ken Murray, "How Doctors Die," *Zócalo Public Square*, http://www.zocalopublicsquare.org/2011/11/30/how-doctors-die/ideas/nexus/.

4. Janet Adamy and Tom McGinty, "The Crushing Cost of Care," *Wall Street Journal* (July 6, 2012); http://www.cms.gov/Research-Statistics-Data-and-Systems/Statistics-Trends-and-Reports/NationalHealthExpendData/downloads/highlights.pdf.

5. L. L. Emanuel et al., "Advance Directives for Medical Care—A Case for Greater Use," *New England Journal of Medicine* 324, no. 13 (1991): 889–895.

6. Christi Parsons and Andrew Zajac, "Senate Committee Scraps Healthcare Provision That Gave Rise to 'Death Panel' Claim," *Los Angeles Times* (August 14, 2009), http://articles.latimes.com/2009/aug/14/nation/na-health-end-of-life14.

7. J. W. Mack et al., "Associations Between End-of-Life Discussion Characteristics and Care Received Near Death: A Prospective Cohort Study," *Journal of Clinical Oncology* 30, no. 35 (2012): 4387–4395.

8. K. E. Covinsky et al., "Communication and Decision Making in Seriously Ill Patients: Findings of the SUPPORT Project," *Journal of the American Geriatric Society* 48 (2000): S187–193.

9. Elisabeth Kübler-Ross, *On Death and Dying* (New York: Scribner, 1969).

10. H. K. Beecher, "The Powerful Placebo," *Journal of the American Medical Association* 159 (1955): 1602–1606.

11. R. Sherman and J. Hickner, "Academic Physicians Use Placebos in Clinical Practice and Believe in the Mind-Body Connection," *Journal of General Internal Medicine* 23, no 1. (2008): 7–10.

12. C. McRae et al., "Effects of Perceived Treatment on Quality of Life and Medical Outcomes in a Double-Blind Placebo Surgery Trial," *Archives of General Psychiatry* 61, no. 4 (2004): 412–420.

13. F. Benedetti and M. Amanzio, "The Placebo Response: How Words and Rituals Change the Patient's Brain," *Patient Education and Counseling* 84 (2011): 413–419; P. Enck and S. Klosterhalfen, "The Story of O—Is Oxytocin the Mediator of the Placebo Response?" *Neurogastroenterology and Motility* 21, no. 4 (2009): 347–350; J. P. Gouin et al., "Marital Behavior, Oxytocin, Vasopressin, and Wound Healing," *Psychoneuroendocrinology* 35, no. 7 (2010): 1082–1090.

14. Michael Balint, *The Doctor, His Patient, and the Illness*, 4th ed. (New York: International Universities Press, 1974), 116.

15. Edward E. Rosenbaum, *The Doctor* (New York: Ivy, 1988), 12.

16. P. Lurie and S. M. Wolfe, "Unethical Trials of Interventions to Reduce Perinatal Transmission of the Human Immunodeficiency Virus in Developing Countries," *New England Journal of Medicine* 337, no. 12 (1997): 853–856.

17. M. Neumann et al., "Can Patient-Provider Interaction Increase the Effectiveness of Medical Treatment or Even Substitute It?—An Exploration on Why and How to Study the Specific Effect of the Provider," *Patient Education and Counseling* 80, no. 3 (2010): 307–314.

18. T. J. Kaptchuk et al., "Placebos Without Deception: A Randomized Controlled Trial in Irritable Bowel Syndrome," *PLoS One* 5, no. 12 (2010): e15591.

19. W. B. Cannon, "Voodoo Death," *American Anthropologist* 44 (1942): 169–181; Paul Enck and Winfried Häuser, "Beware the Nocebo Effect," *New York Times* (August 12, 2012).

20. D. Varelmann et al., "Nocebo-Induced Hyperalgesia During Local Anesthetic Injection," *Anesthesia and Analgesia* 110, no. 3 (2010): 868–870; S. Elsenbruch et al., "How Positive and Negative Expectations Shape the Experience of Visceral Pain: An Experimental Pilot Study in Healthy Women," *Neurogastroenterology and Motility* 24, no. 10 (2012): 914–e460.

3. WHEN WORLDS COLLIDE

1. M. B. Dagnew and M. Damena, "Traditional Child Health Practices in Communicates in Northwest Ethiopia," *Tropical Doctor* 20 (1990): 40–41; A. Rubinstein, "Absence of Uvula in South Sinai Bedouins," *Journal of the American Medical Association* (1970): 323.

2. Preamble to the Constitution of the World Health Organization as adopted by the International Health Conference, New York, June 19–22, 1946; signed on July 22, 1946, by the representatives of sixty-one states and entered into force on April 7, 1948. *Official Records of the World Health Organization* 2:100.

3. R. M. Schwartzstein and L. Adams, "Dyspnea," in *Murray and Nadel Textbook of Respiratory Medicine*, ed. R. J. Mason et al. (Philadelphia: Saunders, 2010), 613.

4. E. H. Kass, "Asymptomatic Infections of the Urinary Tract," Trans Assoc Am Physicians. 1956;69:56–64.

5. M. N. G. Dukes, "Personal View," *British Medical Journal* 5878 (1973): 496; cited in Lynn Payer, *Medicine and Culture: Varieties of Treatment in the United States, England, West Germany, and France*, 2nd ed. (New York: Henry Holt and Company, 1996).

6. Payer, *Medicine and Culture*, 16.

7. David Tuller, "Defining an Illness Is Fodder for Debate," *New York Times* (March 8, 2011).

8. C. F. Norbury and A. Sparks, "Difference or Disorder? Cultural Issues in Understanding Neurodevelopmental Disorders," *Developmental Psychology* 49, no. 1 (2013); http://www.cdc.gov/media/releases/2012/p0329_autism_disorder.html.

9. K. E. Zuckerman et al., "Pediatrician Identification of Latino Children at Risk for Autism Spectrum Disorder," *Pediatrics* 132 (2013): 445–453.

10. Centers for Disease Control and Prevention (CDC), "Prevalence of Autism Spectrum Disorders: Autism and Developmental Disabilities Monitoring Network, United States, 2008," *Morbidity and Mortal Weekly Report* 61, no. 3 (2012).

11. S. N. Visser and C. A. Lesesne, "Mental Health in the United States: Prevalence of Diagnosis and Medication Treatment for Attention-Deficit/Hyperactivity Disorder—United States, 2003," *MMWR Weekly* 54, no. 34 (September 2, 2005): 842–847.

12. K. Takubo et al., "Differences in the Definitions Used for Esophageal and Gastric Diseases in Different Countries: Endoscopic Definition of the Esophagogastric Junction, the Precursor of Barrett's Adenocarcinoma, the Definition of Barrett's Esophagus, and Histologic Criteria for Mucosal Adenocarcinoma or High-Grade Dysplasia," *Digestion* 80, no. 4 (2009): 248–257.

13. V. Prasad et al., "A Decade of Reversal: An Analysis of 146 Contradicted Medical Practices," *Mayo Clinic Proceedings* 88, no. 8 (2013): 790–798.

14. J. Roulson, E. W. Benbow, and P. S. Hasleton, "Discrepancies Between Clinical and Autopsy Diagnosis and the Value of Postmortem Histology: A Metaanalysis and Review," *Histopathology* 47, no. 6 (2005): 551–559; James Meikle, "Inaccurate Cause of Death Recorded for One in Four Patients," *Guardian* (August 10, 2012).

15. Dick Teresi, *The Undead: Organ Harvesting, the Ice-Water Test, Beating-Heart Cadavers—How Medicine Is Blurring the Line Between Life and Death* (New York: Pantheon, 2012).

16. World Health Organization, "Appropriate Technology for Birth," *Lancet* 2, no. 8452 (1985): 436–437. Luz Gibbons et al., "The Global Numbers and Costs of Additionally Needed and Unnecessary Caesarean Sections Performed per Year: Overuse as a Barrier to Universal Coverage," World Health Organization, World Health Report (2010) Background Paper, 30; https://www.cia.gov/library/publications/the-world-factbook/rankorder/2091rank.html; F. C. Notzon, "International Differences in the Use of Obstetric Interventions," *Journal of the American Medical Association* 263 (1990): 3286–3291.

17. World Health Organization, "Appropriate Technology for Birth," *Lancet* 2, no. 8452: 436–437; M. MacDorman, E. Declercq, and F. Menacker, "Recent Trends and P{atterns in Cesarean and Vaginal Birth After Cesarean (VBAC) Deliveries in the United States," *Clinics in Perinatology* 38, no. 2 (2011): 179–192.

18. http://transform.childbirthconnection.org/resources/datacenter/chargeschart/.

19. K. B. Kozhimannil, M. R. Law, and B. A. Virnig, "Cesarean Delivery Rates Vary Tenfold Among US Hospitals; Reducing Variation May Address Quality and Cost Issues," *Health Affairs (Millwood)* 32, no. 3 (2013): 527–535.

20. K. McPherson et al., "Small-Area Variations in the Use of Common Surgical Procedures: An International Comparison of New England, England, and Norway," *New England*

Journal of Medicine 307 (1982): 1310–1314; A. Coulter, K. McPherson, and M. Vessey, "Do British Women Undergo Too Many or Too Few Hysterectomies?" *Social Science and Medicine* 27 (1987): 987–994; G. Lafortune, G. Balestat, and A. Durand, OECD Health Division, "Final Report on Work Package II: Comparing Activities and Performance of the Hospital Sector in Europe: How Many Surgical Procedures Performed as Inpatient and Day Cases?" December 2012, http://www.oecd.org/health/health-systems/Comparing -activities-and-performance-of-the-hospital-sector-in-Europe_Inpatient-and-day-cases -surgical-procedures.pdf.

21. Michel Foucault, *The Birth of the Clinic: An Archeology of Medical Perception*, trans. A. M. Sheridan Smith (New York: Vintage, 1973), 55–56.

22. Merrill Singer and Hans Baer, *Introducing Medical Anthropology*, 2nd ed. (Lanham, Md.: AltaMira, 2012), 84; Daniel Defoe, *A Journal of the Plague Year* (Oxford: Oxford University Press, 2009), 27.

23. Anne Fadiman, *The Spirit Catches You and You Fall Down: A Hmong Child, Her American Doctors, and the Collision of Two Cultures* (New York: Farrar, Strauss and Giroux, 1997), 20, 50.

24. Ibid., 100.

25. J. C. Philp et al., "Complementary and Alternative Medicine Use and Adherence with Pediatric Asthma Treatment," *Pediatrics* 129 (2012): e1148–1154; R. A. Stone et al., "Traditional Practices, Traditional Spirituality, and Alcohol Cessation Among American Indians," *Journal of Studies on Alcohol and Drugs* 67, no. 2 (2006): 236–244.

26. M. Shaked and Y. Bilu, "Grappling with Affliction: Autism in the Jewish Ultraorthodox Community in Israel," *Culture, Medicine, and Psychiatry* 30, no. 1 (2006): 1–27.

27. Ibid.

28. Ibid.

29. Fadiman, *The Spirit Catches You and You Fall Down*, 51.

30. Patricia Leigh Brown, "A Doctor for Disease, a Shaman for the Soul," *New York Times* (September 20, 2009).

31. Jennifer Hirsch and Emily Vasquez, "Immigrant Health: Shamans, 'Soul Calling,' and the Uninsured," http://accessdeniedblog.wordpress.com/2009/12/01/immigrant-health-shamans -%E2%80%98soul-calling%E2%80%99-and-the-uninsured.

32. E. Verlinde et al., "The Social Gradient in Doctor-Patient Communication," *International Journal for Equity in Health* 11 (2012): 12.

33. M. K. Nations and C. M. G. Monte, "'I'm Not Dog, No!' Cries of Resistance Against Cholera Control Campaigns," *Social Science and Medicine* 43 (1996): 1007–1024.

34. Charles L. Briggs, *Stories in the Time of Cholera: Racial Profiling During a Medical Nightmare* (Berkeley: University of California Press, 2003).

35. Paul Farmer, *Partner to the Poor* (Berkeley: University of California Press, 2010), 151.

36. R. H. Gilman et al., "Water Cost and Availability: Key Determinants of Family Hygiene in a Peruvian Shantytown," *American Journal of Public Health* 83 (1993): 1554–1558; R. H. Gilman and P. Skillicorn, "Boiling of Drinking Water: Can a Fuel-Scarce Community Afford It?" *Bulletin of the World Health Organization* 63 (1985): 157–163; D. L. Hatch et al.,

"Epidemic Cholera During Refugee Resettlement in Malawi," *International Journal of Epidemiology* 23, no. 6 (1994): 1292–1299.

4. DISEASE, ILLNESS, AND SICKNESS

1. Arthur Kleinman, *Patients and Healers in the Context of Culture* (Berkeley: University of California Press, 1980), 72.

2. D. Jennings, "The Confusion Between Disease and Illness in Clinical Medicine," *Canadian Medical Association Journal* 135, no. 8 (1986): 865–870.

3. J. A. Barondess, "Disease and Illness—A Crucial Distinction," *American Journal of Medicine* 66, no. 3 (1979): 375–376.

4. Renee Montaigne, "Painful Memories for China's Footbinding Survivors," *National Public Radio Morning Edition* (March 19, 2007), http://www.npr.org/templates/transcript/transcript .php?storyId=8966942; World Health Organization, "Eliminating Female Genital Mutilation: An Interagency Statement," Geneva, 2008.

5. H. Merskey, "Variable Meanings for the Definition of Disease," *Journal of Medicine and Philosophy* 11, no. 3 (1986): 215–232.

6. Oliver Wendell Holmes, *Medical Essays, 1842–1882* (Cambridge, Mass.: Riverside, 1891), 192.

7. James Trostle, *Epidemiology and Culture* (New York: Cambridge University Press, 2005), 11.

8. Ibid., 12.

9. Ibid., 2.

10. S. Dein, "Working with Patients with Religious Beliefs," *Advances in Psychiatric Treatment* 10 (2004): 287–295.

11. D. Mechanic, "The Concept of Illness Behavior," *Journal of Chronic Diseases* 15 (1962): 189–194.

12. C. D. Jenkins, "Group Differences in Perception: A Study of Community Beliefs and Feelings About Tuberculosis," *American Journal of Sociology* 71, no. 4 (1966): 417–429.

13. P. Kelly, "Isolation and Stigma: The Experience of Patients with Active Tuberculosis," *Journal of Community Health Nursing* 16 (1999): 233–241.

14. "Tuberculosis" and "Lung Carcinoma," in *The Merck Manual*, http://www.merckmanuals .com/professional/infectious_diseases/mycobacteria/tuberculosis_tb.html?qt =tuberculosis&alt=sh, http://www.merckmanuals.com/professional/pulmonary_disorders /tumors_of_the_lungs/lung_carcinoma.html?qt=&sc=&alt=.

15. Kelly, "Isolation and Stigma."

16. A. Kleinman, "The Teaching of Clinically Applied Medical Anthropology on a Psychiatric Consultation-Liaison Service," in *Clinically Applied Anthropology: Anthropologists in Health Science Settings*, ed. Noel J. Chrisman and Thomas W. Maretzki (Dordrecht: D. Reidel, 1982), 83–115.

17. Paul Farmer, *Partner to the Poor* (Berkeley: University of California Press, 2010), 33–61.

18. A. Kleinman, *The Illness Narratives: Suffering, Healing, and the Human Condition* (New York: Basic Books, 1988), 4.

19. M. E. Edington, C. S. Sekatane, and S. J. Goldstein, "Patients' Beliefs: Do They Affect Tuberculosis Control? A Study in a Rural District of South Africa," *International Journal of Tuberculosis and Lung Disease* 6 (2002): 1075–1082.

20. Sonia Shah, *The Fever: How Malaria Has Ruled Humankind for 500,000 Years* (New York: Farrar, Straus and Giroux, 2010), 124–125.

21. John Murphy, "Distrust of U.S. Foils Effort to Stop Crippling Disease," *Baltimore Sun* (January 4, 2004).

22. Svea Closser, *Chasing Polio in Pakistan* (Nashville, Tenn.: Vanderbilt University Press, 2010), 180.

23. David M. Oshinsky, *Polio: An American Story* (New York: Oxford University Press, 2005), 70.

24. George Lakoff and Mark Johnson, *Metaphors We Live By* (Chicago: University of Chicago Press, 1980), 185.

25. Christopher Hitchens, *Mortality* (New York: Hachette, 2012), 1.

26. L. J. Kirmayer and A. Young, "Culture and Somatization: Clinical, Epidemiological, and Ethnographic Perspectives," *Psychosomatic Medicine* 60 (1998): 420–430.

27. Mary Robinson, from her lecture "Becoming a Spiritual Generalist" (November 27, 2012).

28. M. Marinker, "Why Make People Patients?" *Journal of Medical Ethics* 1 (1975): 81–84.

29. Thomas Szasz, *The Untamed Tongue: A Dissenting Dictionary* (LaSalle, Ill.: Open Court, 1990), 130.

30. Daniel Defoe, *A Journal of the Plague Year* (Oxford: Oxford University Press, 2009), 14, 198, 36, 68.

31. Dudley Clendinen, "AIDS Spreads Pain and Fear Among Ill and Healthy Alike," *New York Times* (June 17, 1983).

32. B. Weiner, R. P. Perry, and J. Magnusson, "An Attributional Analysis of Reactions to Stigmas," *Journal of Personality and Social Psychology* 55, no. 5 (1988): 738–748.

33. A. Malcolm et al, "HIV-Related Stigmatization: Its Forms and Contexts," *Critical Public Health* 8 (1998): 347–370.

34. Uzodinma Iweala, *Our Kind of People: A Continent's Challenge, a Country's Hope* (New York: HarperCollins, 2012), 67, 70.

35. Susan Sontag, *Illness as Metaphor and AIDS and Its Metaphors* (New York: Picador, 2001), 100.

36. Sandra Ricigliano Dooley, "Pancreatic Cancer Strikes Without Warning," http://em .gmnews.com/news/2011-06-08/Letters/Pancreatic_cancer_strikes_without_warning.html; David Brown, "War Against Cancer Has More Than One Target," *Washington Post* (April 27, 2010); "Texas Center's $3 Billion Plan to Defeat Cancer," *Associated Press* (September 21, 2012), http://healthland.time.com/2012/09/21/texas-cancer-centers-3-billion-plan-to-defeat -cancer/#ixzz276vH98Xe; http://www.conquercancer.org/www.conquercancer.org/Cover .html; Lacy Hilliard, "Mother and Daughter Battle and Survive Cancer Together," *The Tomahawk* (Mountain City, Tenn.), http://www.thetomahawk.com/Detail.php?Cat =HOMEPAGE&ID=59472; Jessie L. Bonner, "Idaho Teen Loses Cancer Fight After Delivering Son," *USA Today* (December 28, 2011); Cynthia Ryan, "Edwards' Brave Fight Was No Doubt Wretched, Too," *USA Today* (December 13, 2010);

37. A. Chapple, S. Ziebland, and A. McPherson, "Stigma, Shame, and Blame Experienced by Patients with Lung Cancer: Qualitative Study," *BMJ* 328, no. 7454 (2004): 1470.

38. M. S. Tracy et al., "Contralateral Prophylactic Mastectomy in Women with Breast Cancer: Trends, Predictors, and Areas for Future Research," *Breast Cancer Research and Treatment* 140, no. 3 (2013): 447–452.

39. L. J. Esserman, I. M. Thompson, and B. Reid, "Overdiagnosis and Overtreatment in Cancer: An Opportunity for Improvement," *Journal of the American Medical Association* (July 29, 2013).

40. L. Gamwell, "Images of Madness: A Portfolio of Nineteenth-Century Women," *Annals of the New York Academy of Sciences* 18, no. 789 (1996): 79–81; J. S. Nairnes, "Neurasthenia (So-called), Hysteria, and Abdominal Section," *British Medical Journal* 2 (1902):1140–1143; Decca Aitkenhead, "The Buzz: How the Vibrator Came to Be" *The Guardian* (September 7, 2012), http://www.guardian.co.uk/lifeandstyle/2012/sep/07/how-the-vibrator-caused-buzz/print.

41. Mark S. Micale, "On the 'Disappearance' of Hysteria: A Study in the Clinical Deconstruction of a Diagnosis," *Isis* 84, no. 3 (1993): 496–526.

42. F. Peterson, "Pelvic Disease: Is It a Cause of Nervous and Mental Affections?" *Journal of the American Medical Association* 32 (1899): 640–642.

43. C. W. Socarides, "Homosexuality and Medicine," *Journal of the American Medical Association* 212 (1970): 1199–1202.

44. http://narth.com/2011/12/narth-practice-guidelines/.

45. William L. Dreikorn, "Sexual Orientation Conversion Therapy: Help or Hindrance?" http://narth.com/docs/helporhind.html.

46. R. L. Spitzer, "Can Some Gay Men and Lesbians Change Their Sexual Orientation? 200 Participants Reporting a Change from Homosexual to Heterosexual Orientation," *Archives of Sexual Behavior* 32 (2003): 403–417.

47. Benedict Carey, "Psychiatry Giant Sorry for Backing Gay 'Cure.'" *New York Times* (May 18, 2012).

48. Neal Broverman, "Arm of the World Health Organization Takes Stance Against Reparative Therapy," *Advocate.com* (May 18, 2012), http://www.advocate.com/health/2012/05/18/world-health-organization-affiliate-discredits-exgay-therapy-and-urges-nations.

49. Erik Eckholm, "California Is First State to Ban Gay 'Cure' for Minors," *New York Times* (September 30, 2012); Madeleine Morgenstern, "California Legislature Passes Nation's First Bill Banning Gay 'Conversion Therapy.'" *Theblaze.com* (September 1, 2012), http://www.theblaze.com/stories/california-legislature-passes-nations-first-bill-banning-gay-conversion-therapy/.

50. M. L. Hatzenbuehler, "The Social Environment and Suicide Attempts in Lesbian, Gay, and Bisexual Youth," *Pediatrics* 127 (2001): 896–903.

51. Richard Bonnie, "Political Abuse of Psychiatry in the Soviet Union and in China: Complexities and Controversies," *Journal of the American Academy of Psychiatry and the Law* 30 (2002): 136–144.

52. Ibid.

53. Walter Reich, "The World of Soviet Psychiatry," *New York Times* (January 30, 1983).

54. Thomas S. Szasz, *The Myth of Mental Illness*, rev. ed. (New York: Harper Collins, 1973), 62–63.

55. Ibid., 260, 268.

56. Matthew Lippman, "The Nazi Doctors Trial and the International Prohibition on Medical Involvement in Torture," *Loyola of Los Angeles International and Comparative Law Review* 15 (1993): 395–441; Robert N. Proctor, "Nazi Doctors, Racial Medicine, and Human Experimentation," in *The Nazi Doctors and the Nuremberg Code: Human Rights in Human Experimentation*, ed. G. J. Annas and M. A. Grodin. (New York: Oxford University Press, 1992), 17–31.

57. Susan M. Reverby, "More Than Fact and Fiction: Cultural Memory and the Tuskegee Syphilis Study," *Hastings Center Report* 31 (2001): 22–28; S. B. Thomas and S. C. Quinn, "The Tuskegee Syphilis Study, 1932 to 1972: Implications for HIV Education and AIDS Risk Education Programs in the Black Community," *American Journal of Public Health* 81 (1991): 1498–1505; Harlon L. Dalton, "AIDS in Blackface," *Daedalus* 3 (1989): 205–227.

58. Jack Ginsburg and Lois Snyder for the American College of Physicians, "Statement of Principles on the Role of Governments in Regulating the Patient-Physician Relationship" (July 2012), http://www.medpagetoday.com/upload/2012/8/10/statement_of_principles .pdf.

59. Charles Fiegl, "Physicians Resist States' Interference in Practice of Medicine," *AMedNews. com* (August 27, 2012), http://www.ama-assn.org/amednews/2012/08/27/gvsc0827.htm.

60. Erik Ekholm, "Healing Process—A Special Report: While Congress Remains Silent, Health Care Transforms Itself," *New York Times* (December 18, 1994).

61. A. C. Kao et al., "The Relationship Between Method of Physician Payment and Patient Trust," *Journal of the American Medical Association* 280 (1998): 1708–1714; D. S. Feldman, D. H. Novack, and E. Gracely, "Effects of Managed Care on Physician-Patient Relationships, Quality of Care, and the Ethical Practice of Medicine: A Physician Survey," *Archives of Internal Medicine* 158 (1998): 1626–1632.

62. Grace-Marie Turner et al., *Why Obamacare Is Wrong for America* (New York: Harper Collins 2012), 10.

63. John O'Shea, MD, "Compromising the Doctor–Patient Relationship: The Impact of the House Health Care Bill," Web Memo, published by *The Heritage Foundation*. July 27, 2009. http://s3.amazonaws.com/thf_media/2009/pdf/wm2563.pdf last accessed 10/30/2012.

64. M. J. Green et al., "Do Gifts from the Pharmaceutical Industry Affect Trust in Physicians?" *Family Medicine* 44 (2012): 323–331; R. V. Gibbons et al., "A Comparison of Physicians' and Patients' Attitudes Toward Pharmaceutical Industry Gifts," *Journal of General Internal Medicine* 13 (1998): 151–154; J. LaPuma et al., "Financial Ties as Part of Informed Consent to Postmarketing Research," *BMJ* 310 (1995): 1660–1661; Kathleen Sharp, *Blood Feud: The Man Who Blew the Whistle on One of the Deadliest Prescription Drugs Ever* (New York: Dutton, 2011); L. I. Iezzoni et al., "Survey Shows That at Least Some Physicians Are Not Always Open or Honest with Patients," *Health Affairs* 31 (2012): 383–391.

65. A. Wazana, "Physicians and the Pharmaceutical Industry: Is a Gift Ever Just a Gift?" *Journal of the American Medical Association* 283 (2000): 373–380.

66. Pew Charitable Trust, "Pew Prescription Project Fact Sheet: Physician Payments Sunshine Provisions in Health Care Reform" (March 23, 2010), http://www.pewhealth.org/upload-edFiles/PHG/Supporting_Items/IB_FS_PPP_Sunshine-fact-sheet.pdf.

67. Thomas Stossel, "Who Paid for Your Doctor's Bagel?" *Wall Street Journal* (January 23, 2012).

5. BODY AND SOUL

1. J. K. Rao et al., "Communication Interventions Make a Difference in Conversations Between Physicians and Patients: A Systematic Review of the Evidence," *Medical Care* 45, no. 4 (2007): 340–349; C. Lagan et al., "Evaluation of an Interprofessional Clinician-Patient Communication Workshop Utilizing Standardized Patient Methodology," *Journal of Surgical Education* 70, no. 1 (2013): 95–103; N. K. Ali, "Are We Training Residents to Communicate with Low Health Literacy Patients?" *Journal of Community Hospital Internal Medicine Perspectives* 2, no. 4 (2013).

2. C. S. Skinner et al., "Use of and Reactions to a Tailored CD-ROM Designed to Enhance Oncologist-Patient Communication: The SCOPE Trial Intervention," *Patient Education and Counseling* 77 (2009): 90–96; D. Thew et al., "The Deaf Strong Hospital Program: A Model of Diversity and Inclusion Training for First-Year Medical Students," *Academic Medicine* 87 (2012): 1496–500; S. Kripalani et al., "Development and Evaluation of a Medication Counseling Workshop for Physicians: Can We Improve on 'Take Two Pills and Call Me in the Morning'?" *Medical Education Online* 16 (2011); Laura Landro, "The Talking Cure for Health Care," *Wall Street Journal* (April 8, 2013).

3. V. A. Jackson and A. L. Back, "Teaching Communication Skills Using Role-Play: An Experience-Based Guide for Educators," *Journal of Palliative Medicine* 14 (2011): 775–780; J. O. Schell et al., "Communication Skills Training for Dialysis Decision-Making and End-of-Life Care in Nephrology," *Clinical Journal of the American Society of Nephrology* 8, no. 4 (2013): 675–680.

4. E. C. Meyer et al., "An Interdisciplinary, Family-Focused Approach to Relational Learning in Neonatal Intensive Care," *Journal of Perinatology* 31, no. 3 (2011): 212–219.

5. E. C. Meyer et al., "Difficult Conversations: Improving Communication Skills and Relational Abilities in Health Care," *Pediatric Critical Care Medicine* 10, no. 3 (2009): 352–359; J. M. Clayton et al., "Intensive Communication Skills Teaching for Specialist Training in Palliative Medicine: Development and Evaluation of an Experiential Workshop," *Journal of Palliative Medicine* 15, no. 5 (2012): 585–591.

6. http://www.cancer.org/cancer/leukemiainchildren/overviewguide/childhood-leukemia-overview-survival-rates.

7. G. L. Engel, "The Need for a New Medical Model: A Challenge for Biomedicine," *Science* 196 (1977): 129–136.

6. RECONCILING DIFFERENT WORLDVIEWS

1. J. S. Taylor, "The Story Catches You and You Fall Down," *Medical Anthropology Quarterly* 17, no. 2 (2003).
2. J. S. Taylor, "Confronting 'Culture' in Medicine's 'Culture of No Culture.'" *Academic Medicine* 78 (2003): 555–559.
3. Anne Fadiman, *The Spirit Catches You and You Fall Down: A Hmong Child, Her American Physicians, and the Collision of Two Cultures* (New York: Farrar, Strauss and Giroux, 1997), 76.
4. Ibid., 276.
5. Thomas Szasz, *The Second Sin* (Garden City, N.Y.: Anchor, 1973), 115.
6. M. Tervalon and J. Murray-García, "Cultural Humility Versus Cultural Competence: A Critical Distinction in Defining Physician Training Outcomes in Multicultural Education," *Journal of Health Care for the Poor and Underserved* 9, no. 2 (1998): 117–125.
7. Elizabeth Kübler-Ross, *On Death and Dying* (New York: Scribner, 1969).
8. P. Ashurst, "On Listening to the Patient: Commentary on . . . The Long Case Is Dead," *The Psychiatrist* 31 (2007): 446–447.
9. A. R. Green et al., "Implicit Bias Among Physicians and Its Prediction of Thrombolysis Decisions for Black and White Patients," *Journal of General Internal Medicine* 22, no. 9 (2007): 1231–1238.
10. M. Campesino et al., "Perceived Discrimination and Ethnic Identity Among Breast Cancer Survivors," *Oncology Nursing Forum* 39, no. 2 (2012): E91–100.
11. L. S. Rintamaki et al., "Male Patient Perceptions of HIV Stigma in Health Care Contexts," *AIDS Patient Care and STDs* 21 (2007): 956–969.
12. J. J. Kinsler et al., "The Effect of Perceived Stigma from a Health Care Provider on Access to Care Among a Low-Income HIV-Positive Population," *AIDS Patient Care and STDs* 21, no. 8 (2007): 584–592.
13. C. L. Olson, H. D. Schumaker, and B. P. Yawn, "Overweight Women Delay Medical Care," *Archives of Family Medicine* 3, no. 10 (1994): 888–892.
14. C. C. Wee et al., "Screening for Cervical and Breast Cancer: Is Obesity an Unrecognized Barrier to Preventive Care?" *Annals of Internal Medicine* 132, no. 9 (2000): 697–704; N. K. Amy et al., "Barriers to Routine Gynecological Cancer Screening for White and African-American obese women," *International Journal of Obesity* (London) 30, no. 1 (2006): 147–155.
15. David Katz, "When Physicians Judge Their Obese Patients," *Huffington Post* (March 16, 2011), http://www.huffingtonpost.com/david-katz-md/obesity-of-blame-and-sham_b_834937.html.
16. B. M. Parker et al., "The Test of Functional Health Literacy in Adults: A New Instrument for Measuring Patients' Literacy Skills," *Journal of General Internal Medicine* 10 (1995): 537–541.
17. D. H. Howard, J. Gazmararian, and R. M. Parker, "The Impact of Low Health Literacy on the Medical Costs of Medicare Managed Care Enrollees," *American Journal of Medicine* 118, no. 4 (2005): 371–377; S. E. Mitchell et al., "Health Literacy and 30-Day Postdischarge

Hospital Utilization," *Journal of Health Communication* 17, suppl. 3 (2012): 325–338; C. Y. Osborn et al., "Health Literacy Explains Racial Disparities in Diabetes Medication Adherence," *Journal of Health Communication* 16, suppl. 3 (2011): 268–278; N. A. Hardie et al., "Health Literacy and Health Care Spending and Utilization in a Consumer-Driven Health Plan," *Journal of Health Communication* 16, suppl. 3 (2011): 308–321; C. K. Powell and S. Kripalani, "Brief Report: Resident Recognition of Low Literacy as a Risk Factor in Hospital Readmission," *Journal of General Internal Medicine* 20, no. 11 (2005): 1042–1044.

18. V. L. Welch, J. B. VanGeest, and R. Caskey, "Time, Costs, and Clinical Utilization of Screening for Health Literacy: A Case Study Using the Newest Vital Sign (NVS) Instrument," *Journal of the American Board of Family Medicine* 24, no. 3 (2011): 281–289.

19. B. D. Weiss and R. Palmer, "Relationship Between Health Care Costs and Very Low Literacy Skills in a Medically Needy and Indigent Medicaid Population," *Journal of the American Board of Family Practice* 17, no. 1 (2004): 44–47.

20. Christopher Hitchens, *Mortality* (New York: Hachette, 2012), 67.

21. Pam Belluck, *Island Practice: Cobblestone Rash, Underground Tom, and Other Adventures of a Nantucket Physician* (New York: Public Affairs, 2012), 44.

22. E. G. Laforet, "The Fiction of Informed Consent," *Journal of the American Medical Association* 235 (1978): 1579–1585.

23. Irwin Press, "Witch Physician's Legacy: Some Anthropological Implications for the Practice of Clinical Medicine," in *Clinically Applied Anthropology*, ed. N. J. Chrisman and T. W. Maretzki (Dordrecht: Reidel, 1982), 179–198.

7. MAKING IT STICK

1. *Monty Python and The Holy Grail* (1975), directed by Terry Gilliam and Terry Jones.

2. Centers for Disease Control and Prevention (CDC), "Vital Signs: Overdoses of Prescription Opioid Pain Relievers—United States, 1999–2008," *MMWR Morbidity and Mortality Weekly Report* 60, no. 43 (2011): 1487; C. M. Jones, K. A. Mack, and L. J. Paulozzi, "Pharmaceutical Overdose Deaths, United States, 2010," *Journal of the American Medical Association* 309, no. 7 (2013): 657–659; National Institute on Drug Abuse Research Report Series, "Prescription Drugs: Abuse and Addiction," http://www.drugabuse.gov/sites/default/files/rrprescription.pdf.

3. P. G. Gibson et al., "Self-Management Education and Regular Practitioner Review for Adults with Asthma," *Cochrane Database of Systematic Reviews* 1 (2003): CD001117.

4. S. Lo, D. L. Stuenkel, and L. Rodriguez, "The Impact of Diagnosis-Specific Discharge Instructions on Patient Satisfaction," *Journal of PeriAnesthesia Nursing* 24, no. 3 (2009): 156–162.

5. A. D. Muthusamy et al., "Supplemental Written Information Improves Prenatal Counseling: A Randomized Trial," *Pediatrics* 129, no. 5 (2012): e1269–1274; T. Fayers et al., "Impact of Written and Photographic Instruction Sheets on Patient Behavior After Cataract Surgery," *Journal of Cataract and Refractive Surgery* 35, no. 15 (2009): 1739–1743; R. Negarandeh et al.,

"Teach Back and Pictorial Image Educational Strategies on Knowledge About Diabetes and Medication/Dietary Adherence Among Low Health Literate Patients with Type 2 Diabetes," *Primary Care Diabetes* (November 26, 2012), doi:pii: S1751–9918(12)00221–5; S. Choi et al., "The Effectiveness of Mobile Discharge Instruction Videos (MDIVs) in Communicating Discharge Instructions to Patients with Lacerations or Sprains," *Southern Medical Journal* 102, no. 3 (2009): 239–247.

6. K. D. Keith et al., "Emergency Department Revisits," *Annals of Emergency Medicine* 18, no. 9 (1989): 964–968; K. G. Engel et al., "Patient Understanding of Emergency Department Discharge Instructions: Where Are Knowledge Deficits Greatest?" *Academic Emergency Medicine* 19, no. 9 (2012): E1035–1044; D. M. McCarthy et al., "Emergency Department Discharge Instructions: Lessons Learned Through Developing New Patient Education Materials," *Emergency Medicine International* (2012), doi: 10.1155/2012/306859.

7. A. Vashi and K. V. Rhodes, "'Sign Right Here and You're Good to Go': A Content Analysis of Audiotaped Emergency Department Discharge Instructions," *Annals of Emergency Medicine* 57 (2011): 315–322; K. G. Engel et al., "Patient Comprehension of Emergency Department Care and Instructions: Are Patients Aware of When They do Not Understand?" *Annals of Emergency Medicine* 53, no. 5 (2009): 454–461.

8. J. W. Showalter et al., "Effect of Standardized Electronic Discharge Instructions on Postdischarge Hospital Utilization," *Journal of General Internal Medicine* 26, no. 7 (2011): 718–723; M. White et al., "Is 'Teach-Back' Associated with Knowledge Retention and Hospital Readmission in Hospitalized Heart Failure Patients?" *Journal of Cardiovascular Nursing* 28, no. 2 (2013): 137–146; H. S. Yin et al., "Readability, Suitability, and Characteristics of Asthma Action Plans: Examination of Factors That May Impair Understanding," *Pediatrics* 131 (2013): e116–126.

9. A. J. Jager and M. K. Wynia, "Who Gets a Teach-Back? Patient-Reported Incidence of Experiencing a Teach Back," *Journal of Health Communication* 17 (2012): 294–302.

10. Ibid.; V. L. Welch, J. B. VanGeest, and R. Caskey, "Time, Costs, and Clinical Utilization of Screening for Health Literacy: A Case Study Using the Newest Vital Sign (NVS) Instrument," *Journal of the American Board of Family Medicine* 24, no. 3 (2011): 281–289.

11. D. M. Tarn et al., "How Much Time Does It Take to Prescribe a New Medication?" *Patient Education and Counseling* 72, no. 2 (2008): 311–319.

12. Plastic tubes into which aerosolized medications are released, which enables the medications to be delivered to the lungs much more easily and effectively.

13. A. L. Buchanan et al., "Barriers to Medication Adherence in HIV-Infected Children and Youth Based on Self- and Caregiver Report," *Pediatrics* 129 (2012): e1244–1251.

14. S. Rollnick, W. R. Miller, and C. C. Butler, *Motivational Interviewing in Health Care* (New York: Guilford, 2008); W. R. Miller and G. S. Rose, "Toward a Theory of Motivational Interviewing," *American Psychologist* 64, no. 6 (2009): 527–537.

15. B. Sleath et al., "Communication During Pediatric Asthma Visits and Self-Reported Asthma Medication Adherence," *Pediatrics* 130 (2012): 627–633.

16. N. K. Arora and C. A. McHorney, "Patient Preferences for Medical Decision Making: Who Really Wants to Participate?" *Medical Care* 38, no. 3 (2000): 335–341.

17. R. M. Epstein, "Whole Mind and Shared Mind in Clinical Decision-Making," *Patient Education and Counseling* 90 (2013): 200–206.

18. K. Cox et al., "Patients' Involvement in Decisions About Medicines: GPs' Perceptions of Their Preferences," *British Journal of General Practice* 57, no. 543 (2007): 777–784.

19. F. Légaré et al., "Training Family Physicians in Shared Decision-Making to Reduce the Overuse of Antibiotics in Acute Respiratory Infections: A Cluster Randomized Trial," *Canadian Medical Association Journal* 184, no. 13 (2012): E726–734.

20. D. Veroff, A. Marr, and D. E. Wennberg, "Enhanced Support for Shared Decision Making Reduced Costs of Care for Patients with Preference-Sensitive Conditions," *Health Affairs* (Millwood) 32, no. 2 (2013): 285–293; A. G. Fiks et al., "Shared Decision-Making and Health Care Expenditures Among Children with Special Health Care Needs," *Pediatrics* 129, no. 1 (2012): 99–107; D. Arterburn et al., "Introducing Decision Aids at Group Health Was Linked to Sharply Lower Hip and Knee Surgery Rates and Costs," *Health Affairs* (Millwood) 31, no. 9 (2012): 2094–2104.

21. G. A. Lin et al., "An Effort to Spread Decision Aids in Five California Primary Care Practices Yielded Low Distribution, Highlighting Hurdles," *Health Affairs* (Millwood) 32, no. 2 (2013): 311–320; M. W. Friedberg et al., "A Demonstration of Shared Decision Making in Primary Care Highlights Barriers to Adoption and Potential Remedies," *Health Affairs* (Millwood) 32, no. 2 (2013): 268–275.

22. http://www.aana.com/ceandeducation/becomeacrna/Pages/Qualifications-and-Capabilities -of-the-Certified-Registered-Nurse-Anesthetist-.aspx.

23. R. M. Epstein et al., "Patient-Centered Communication and Diagnostic Testing," *Annals of Family Medicine* 3 (2005): 415–421.

24. L. Block et al., "In the Wake of the 2003 and 2011 Duty Hours Regulations, How Do Internal Medicine Interns Spend Their Time?" *Journal of General Internal Medicine* (2013), PubMed PMID: 23595927.

25. M. Tai-Seale, T. G. McGuire, and W. Zhang, "Time Allocation in Primary Care Office Visits," *Health Services Research* 42, no. 5 (2007): 1871–1894.

26. Michelle Andrews, "Group Medical Appointments May Help Ease Growing Demands on Healthcare System," *Washington Post* (March 18, 2013).

27. Gardiner Harris, "Talk Doesn't Pay, So Psychiatry Turns to Drug Therapy," *New York Times* (March 5, 2011); M. L. van Hees et al., "The Effectiveness of Individual Interpersonal Psychotherapy as a Treatment for Major Depressive Disorder in Adult Outpatients: A Systematic Review," *BMC Psychiatry* (January 11, 2013): 13–22; C. Ruengorn et al., "Factors Related to Suicide Attempts Among Individuals with Major Depressive Disorder," *International Journal of General Medicine* 5 (2012): 323–330.

28. J. A. Sakowski et al., "Peering Into the Black Box: Billing and Insurance Activities in a Medical Group," *Health Affairs* (Millwood) 28, no. 4 (2009): w544–554.

29. E. Doerr et al., "Between-Visit Workload in Primary Care," *Journal of General Internal Medicine* 25, no. 12 (2010): 1289–1292.

30. L. T. Kohn et al., eds., *To Err Is Human: Building a Safer Health System* (Washington, D.C.: National Academy Press, 2000).

31. Ibid., 1–16.

32. Committee on Identifying and Preventing Medication Errors Board on Health Care Services, *Preventing Medication Errors*, ed. Philip Aspden et al., Institute of Medicine of the National Academies (Washington, D.C.: National Academy Press, 2006).

33. R. Hillestad and J. H. Bigelow, "Health Information Technology: Can HIT Lower Costs and Improve Quality?" (2005), http://www.rand.org/content/dam/rand/pubs/research _briefs/2005/RAND_RB9136.pdf.

34. Centers for Medicare & Medicaid Services, "Fact Sheet: Electronic Health Records—At a Glance: Achieving Rapid Adoption and Meaningful Use" (July 13, 2010), http://www .ncdhhs.gov/dma/ehr/EHRFactSheet.pdf.

35. C. J. Hsaio et al., "Electronic Medical Record/Electronic Health Record Systems of Office-Based Physicians: United States, 2009 and Preliminary 2010 State Estimates" (December 2010), http://www.cdc.gov/nchs/data/hestat/emr_ehr_09/emr_ehr_09.pdf.

36. M. Reed et al., "Outpatient Electronic Health Records and the Clinical Care and Outcomes of Patients with Diabetes Mellitus," *Annals of Internal Medicine* 157 (2012): 482–489; D. O'Reilly et al., "The Economics of Health Information Technology in Medication Management: A Systemic Review of Economic Evaluations," *Journal of the American Medical Informatics Association* 19 (2012): 423–438; R. Abelson et al., "Medicare Bills Rise as Records Turn Electronic," *New York Times* (September 21, 2012); A. L. Kellerman and S. S. Jones, "What Will It Take to Achieve the as-yet Unfulfilled Promises of Health Information Technology?" *Health Affairs* 32 (2013): 63–68.

37. Leora Horowitz, "A Shortcut to Wasted Time," *New York Times* (November 22, 2012).

38. Anne Marie Valinoti, "Physician, Steel Thyself for Electronic Records," *Wall Street Journal* (October 23, 2012).

39. G. Makoul, R. L. Curry, and P. C. Tang, "The Use of Electronic Medical Records: Communication Patterns in Outpatient Encounters," *Journal of the American Medical Informatics Association* 8 (2001): 610–615.

40. A. S. O'Malley, G. R. Cohen, and J. M. Grossman, "Electronic Medical Records and Communication with Other Patients and Other Clinicians: Are We Talking Less?" Center for Studying Health System Change Issue Brief 131 (April 2012), http://www.hschange.com /CONTENT/1125/1125.pdf.

41. Ibid.; E. Rouf et al., "Computers in the Exam Room: Differences in Physician-Patient Interaction May Be Due to Physician Experience," *Journal of General Internal Medicine* 22, no. 1 (2007): 43–48; R. Frankel et al., "Effects of Exam-Room Computing on Clinician-Patient Communication," *Journal of General Internal Medicine* 20 (2005): 677–682.

42. R. Frankel et al., "Effects of Exam-Room Computing."

43. P. E. Kummervold and J. A. Johnsen, "Physician Response Time When Communicating with Patients Over the Internet," *Journal of Medical Internet Research* 13 (2001): e79.

44. M. K. Mittal et al., "Assessment of E-mail Communication Skills of Rheumatology Fellows: A Pilot Study," *Journal of the American Medical Informatics Association* 17 (2010): 702–706.

45. M. E. Wilcox and N. K. Adhikari, "The Effect of Telemedicine in Critically Ill Patients: Systematic Review and Meta-Analysis," *Critical Care* 16, no. 4 (2012): R127.

46. J. Lehrner et al., "Ambient Odor of Orange in a Dental Office Reduces Anxiety and Improves Mood in Female Patients," *Physiology and Behavior* 71, no. 1–2 (2000): 83–86.

47. G. Rice, J. Ingram, and J. Mizan, "Enhancing a Primary Care Environment: A Case Study of Effects on Patients and Staff in a Single General Practice," *British Journal of General Practice* 58, no. 552 (2008): 465–470.

48. J. M. McGrath, N. H. Arar, and J. A. Pugh, "The Influence of Electronic Medical Record Usage on Nonverbal Communication in the Medical Interview," *Health Informatics Journal* 13, no. 2 (2007): 105–118.

49. J. E. Swan, L. D. Richardson, and J. D. Hutton, "Do Appealing Hospital Rooms Increase Patient Evaluations of Physicians, Nurses, and Hospital Services?" *Health Care Management Review* 28, no. 3 (2003): 254–264.

50. Lindsay Abrams, "How Much Should Be Spent Beautifying Hospitals?" *TheAtlantic.com* (March 4, 2013), http://www.theatlantic.com/health/archive/2013/03/how-much-should-be-spent-beautifying-hospitals/273294/; R. S. Ulrich et al., "The Environment's Impact on Stress," in *Improving Healthcare with Better Building Design*, ed. Sara O. Marberry (Chicago: Health Administration Press, 2006), 37–61.

51. D. K. Hamilton and R. D. Orr, "Cultural Transformation and Design," in *Improving Healthcare with Better Building Design*, ed. Sara O. Marberry (Chicago: Health Administration Press, 2006), 146–147.

52. http://www.healthdesign.org.

8. PUTTING IT ALL TOGETHER: CREATING A BETTER CLINICAL ENCOUNTER

1. C. A. Feddock et al., "Is Time Spent with the Physician Associated with Parent Dissatisfaction Due to Long Waiting Times?" *Evaluation and the Health Professions* 33, no. 2 (2010): 216–225.

2. M. H. Oermann, "Effects of Educational Intervention in Waiting Room on Patient Satisfaction," *Journal of Ambulatory Care Management* 26, no. 2 (2003): 150–158.

3. L. Warner et al., "Safe in the City Study Group. Effect of a Brief Video Intervention on Incident Infection Among Patients Attending Sexually Transmitted Disease Clinics," *PLoS Med* 5, no. 6 (2008): e135; M. Trent et al., "Results of a Randomized Controlled Trial of a Brief Behavioral Intervention for Pelvic Inflammatory Disease in Adolescents," *Journal of Pediatric and Adolescent Gynecology* 23, no. 2 (2010): 96–101.

4. A. W. Armstrong et al., "Portable Video Media for Presenting Informed Consent and Wound Care Instructions for Skin Biopsies: A Randomized Controlled Trial," *British Journal of Dermatology* 163, no. 5 (2010): 1014–1019; A. N. Shukla et al., "Informed Consent for Cataract Surgery: Patient Understanding of Verbal, Written, and Videotaped Information," *Journal of Cataract and Refractive Surgery* 38, no. 1 (2012): 80–84.

5. B. M. Kuehn, "More Than One-Third of U.S. Individuals Use the Internet to Self-Diagnose," *Journal of the American Medical Association* 309 (2013): 756–757.

6. http://www.ahrq.gov/patients-consumers/patient-involvement/ask-your-doctor/index .html.

7. http://www.ahrq.gov/apps/qb/.

8. A. Mehrabian and S. R. Ferris, "Inference of Attitudes from Nonverbal Communication in Two Channels," *Journal of Counseling Psychology* 31 (1967): 248–252.

9. L. Marcinowicz, J. Konstantynowicz, and C. Godlewski, "Patients' Perceptions of GP Nonverbal Communication: A Qualitative Study," *British Journal of General Practice* 60 (2012): 83–87.

10. Danielle Ofri, *What Doctors Feel* (Boston: Beacon, 2013), 34–35.

11. L. Marcinowicz, J. Konstantynowicz, and C. Godlewski, "Patients' Perceptions of GP Nonverbal Communication."

12. K. J. Swayden et al., "Effect of Sitting Versus Standing on Perception of Provider Time at Bedside: A Pilot Study," *Patient Education and Counseling* 86, no. 2 (2012): 166–171.

13. Michael Balint, *The Doctor, His Patient, and the Illness*, 4th ed. (New York: International Universities Press, 1974).

14. Joanna C. Schwartz, "Learning from Litigation," *New York Times* (May 16, 2013).

INDEX